Forget the Facelift

Forget the Facelift

Turn Back the Clock with
a Revolutionary Program
for Ageless Skin

Doris J. Day, M.D.
with Sondra Forsyth

Avery
a member of Penguin Group (USA) Inc. • New York

Published by the Penguin Group

Penguin Group (USA) Inc., 375 Hudson Street, New York, New York 10014, USA •
Penguin Group (Canada), 90 Eglinton Avenue East, Suite 700, Toronto, Ontario M4P 2Y3, Canada
(a division of Pearson Penguin Canada Inc.) • Penguin Books Ltd, 80 Strand, London WC2R 0RL, England •
Penguin Ireland, 25 St Stephen's Green, Dublin 2, Ireland (a division of Penguin Books Ltd) •
Penguin Group (Australia), 250 Camberwell Road, Camberwell, Victoria 3124,
Australia (a division of Pearson Australia Group Pty Ltd) • Penguin Books India Pvt Ltd,
11 Community Centre, Panchsheel Park, New Delhi–110 017, India • Penguin Group (NZ),
Cnr Airborne and Rosedale Roads, Albany, Auckland 1310, New Zealand (a division of
Pearson New Zealand Ltd) • Penguin Books (South Africa) (Pty) Ltd, 24 Sturdee Avenue,
Rosebank, Johannesburg 2196, South Africa

Penguin Books Ltd, Registered Offices: 80 Strand, London WC2R 0RL, England

First trade paperback edition 2006

Photos on page 149 courtesy Dr. Michael Ghalili, www.dentistnyc.com
Photos on pages 226 and 242 courtesy Allergan, Inc.
Photos on pages 248 and 249 courtesy Q-Med AB

The Library of Congress catalogued the hardcover edition as follows:

Day, Doris J.
Forget the facelift: turn back the clock with Dr. Day's revolutionary four-step
program for ageless skin/Doris J. Day with Sondra Forsyth.
p.   cm
Includes index.
ISBN 1-58333-232-4
ISBN 1-58333-261-8 (paperback edition)
1. Skin—Care and hygiene. 2. Beauty, Personal. I. Forsyth, Sondra. II. Title.
RL87.D39   2005   2005041209
646.7'26—dc22

Printed in the United States of America
1   3   5   7   9   10   8   6   4   2

Book design by Lovedog Studio

Neither the authors nor the publisher is engaged in rendering professional advice or services to the individual
reader. The ideas, procedures, and suggestions contained in this book are not intended as a substitute for consult-
ing with your physician. All matters regarding your health require medical supervision. Neither the authors nor the
publisher shall be liable or responsible for any loss, injury, or damage allegedly arising from any information or sug-
gestion in this book. The opinions expressed in this book represent the personal views of the authors and not of
the publisher.

While the authors have made every effort to provide accurate telephone numbers and Internet addresses at the time
of publication, neither the publisher nor the authors assume any responsibility for errors, or for changes that occur after
publication. Further, the publisher does not have any control over and does not assume any responsibility for author or
third-party websites or their content.

Most Avery books are available at special quantity discounts for bulk purchase for sales promotions, premiums,
fund-raising, and educational needs. Special books or book excerpts also can be created to fit specific needs. For details, write Penguin Group (USA) Inc. Special Markets, 375 Hudson Street, New York, NY 10014.

For my sister, Adriane (1963–1978).
May this book be a lasting testimony to the beautiful person
she was, inside and out.

For my daughter, Sabrina Adriane.
She is my gift and my inspiration. I offer this gift to her.

Acknowledgments

I want to thank my patients, not only because they encouraged me to write this book but also because they generously shared inspiring entries from their journals.

Deep gratitude also goes to my husband, Michael, for his unfailing support during the writing process and for his seemingly innate and unwavering view of me as the person I continually aspire to become. Sincere thanks also go to my daughter, Sabrina, who read many sections of the book and offered valuable insights, and who continues to amaze me with a far more profound understanding of the world than would seem possible for one so young. As for my son, Andrew, he deserves hugs and sincere appreciation for his encouragements of my efforts, and for cheerfully giving up some quality time with me so that I could meet my deadlines.

A special thank-you goes to my parents, Mansour and Shekoufeh, for their love and wisdom while I found my path in life. In many ways, this book's core message traces back to their rich heritage.

My literary agent, Jessica Papin, of Dystel and Goderich Literary Management, had faith in this project from the very beginning, and her interest never flagged for a minute. I feel fortunate that Jessica came to agenting after a career as a book editor. She often wore her editor's hat while poring over my pages and that fact vastly improved my work. Not long after I submitted the manuscript to my editor, Jessica left to start a new chapter of her life with her husband in their posts at the American University of Cairo. I was honored that Jessica gave my project to Jane Dystel. Jane brought great expertise, experience, and enthusiasm to the final stages of my work on this book.

I am deeply grateful to Megan Newman, publisher of Avery books, for recognizing the importance of this project and staying involved every step of the way. Thanks also go to Dara Stewart for her astute editing of the book, and to all the excellent editors at Avery who had a hand in making these pages the best they could possibly be.

I am indebted to the talented members of the product development team at Good Skin, a division of the Estée Lauder Companies, for their cooperation in getting the word out about this book.

Finally, I want to express my deepest thanks to my coauthor, Sondra Forsyth. Not only was she a pleasure to work with from start to finish but her extensive background in publishing and the arts, combined with my knowledge of anti-aging strategies for the skin, made us the perfect team to deliver just the book that would express my vision for a better, fulfilling, rewarding life—or even one in which we are able to appreciate the good around us and within us, and to maximize our potential, starting with beautiful skin.

Contents

Step 3: The Ageless Skin Diet and Exercise Program

Step 4: Ageless Skin Without Surgery: Botox and Beyond

Introduction:
Beauty Isn't Only
Skin-Deep

I'm going to share with you the secrets of my one-of-a-kind program that promotes both ageless skin and a renewed sense of overall well-being. I developed my program because the skin is the window of all health—physical, emotional, psychological, and spiritual. Even the most up-to-date topical creams and skin treatments won't be truly effective unless you also address related issues that impact how your skin looks. Your skin, after all, is not just a surface—although plenty of people, including a lot of physicians, think of it that way.

Once, when I was speaking to my daughter's third-grade class about dermatology, I asked for the children's definitions of "skin." Many hands shot up, and I called on an earnest-looking boy who said confidently, "Skin wraps us up so our bones don't fall on the floor." Not a bad answer, especially from an eight-year-old. But skin is much, much more than "wrapping." That's why, when you make a conscious decision to have skin that is healthier and more vibrant, you have to look both inside and out in order to get the best results.

That's also why I'm a full-service, solutions-oriented dermatologist. One of my patients, Lucille, dubbed me with that title. As she put it: "You're a combination of doctor, mom, therapist, girlfriend, cheerleader, fashion consultant, beauty adviser, nutritionist, and personal trainer. I could get Botox from any board-certified physician in the phone book. But you do so much more than erase wrinkles. You've changed my life."

Now I'm going to change yours. I know my program will work for you because I see results every day in my office on New York's Upper East Side. I get an intense swell of energy from witnessing the remarkable changes in my patients' skin. As they follow my program, they literally look younger by the day. A key factor in this little miracle is that they not only learn excellent skin care but also start to look at their circumstances from a positive point of view and to take control of their lives. After all, if a woman comes in with a deep frown on her face, erasing that furrow with Botox isn't going to eradicate whatever problems caused the negative facial expression in the first place, so the problem may well come back. For this reason, along with a treatment such as Botox, I teach my patients to work on themselves spiritually and physically, so they will need fewer Botox treatments in the future. The mind and the body are not so much a connection as they are a continuum. The effect of the one on the other is subtle, profound, and critical in the appearance and health of the skin.

I know this from personal experience. I learned about loss and grief firsthand at the age of fifteen, when my beloved and previously healthy fourteen-year-old sister died of cancer. As a result, I have become a better observer of other people's emotional pain. I understand, from my own personal experiences, not to mention from my education and my practice as a physician who takes care of patients every day, that we sometimes punish ourselves with unhealthy lifestyle choices. I did that by suffering for years in private. I gained more than fifty pounds. I made poor choices in the care of my body. It was as if I were standing at the edge of what seemed like a black hole that was deep and endless pain and misery. It seemed so easy, and even almost natural, to fall in, but I knew if I allowed myself to do that, there would be no way out. I had to find a way to back away from the edge of that black hole and get to a better place.

Finally, as an undergrad at Columbia University, I not only came to terms with what I was doing to myself but also made a decision that I was going to live a life like no other, that I had an obligation to do so, and that it was okay to be happy and alive. I knew that, for me, the way forward was to accept that my pain was now a part of me but did not have to be all of me. I knew that I needed to allow my pain to help me show others how much life has to offer. I knew, too, that my path in life was to try to be a better person and to make a difference, in my own way, in order to honor the beautiful and bright person that my sister had been. I came to understand that every day is a gift and an opportunity to love ourselves and to show our love to those who matter most to us. I had a lot of work to do, and through it I gained a point of view that has given me a deeper understanding of myself and what my life was about. Things take on a different perspective when you miss someone so much it hurts and you know you will never be able to see the person again or touch her again. You don't want to overlook any opportunity to revel in the love and life that surround you, and you realize that being as healthy as possible is essential.

That realization was the spark that inspired me to become a physician. However, my father also made me want to become a doctor. He taught me by example that being a physician is not just a job but a calling, and that it is not simply what you do but who you are.

My father is a physician whose specialty is anesthesiology. From the time I was a little girl, he took me with him on his rounds and talked to me about why he felt it was so important for him to get to know his patients before deciding on the best form of anesthesia for each case. He taught me to respect the inextricable connections between the mind, the body, and the soul. He showed me that the art of medicine is best taught through apprenticeship. Watching him with his patients gave me more than I could have learned from any book. The confidence and calm he instilled in his patients just by talking to them were a powerful lesson for me. He was born in Iran, and Middle Eastern philosophy profoundly influenced his way of practicing medicine in the West. I was privileged to be heir to that, and then to rediscover its value and make it my own.

I am also very fortunate to have a husband who is a dentist who had been in practice for several years before I met him. When his patients told me about his gentleness, caring, and sensitivity, I could see not only that there are doctors in all fields of medicine who consider it an art and a way of life that brings personal satisfaction and fulfillment through doing for others but also that I was making a great choice for a husband, partner in life, and father of my children.

All that I have just shared with you about my personal journey, along with my travels and education, has helped to shape my mind/body/spirit approach to rejuvenating the skin. However, I don't like to have the adjective "holistic" applied to my program. Even though I emphasize the absolute truth and importance of the mind/body/spirit connection, I don't espouse a method that's simply contrarian or "touchy-feely," as do many people who call themselves practitioners of holistic medicine. I am first and foremost a physician. I do not advocate what is often called "alternative" medicine, to the exclusion of traditional Western medicine. My program is based on solid medical evidence, not hearsay or experimental notions. It was in medical school that I realized that the skin has the ability to rejuvenate itself. Wrinkles, brown spots, and changes in texture are not an inevitable part of the natural aging process. They are actually signs of distress that can be reversed. Also, during my psychology rotation I became fascinated with the way the mind can affect the body. For a while, I considered becoming a psychiatrist. However, I observed that although people often hesitate to get professional help for mental and emotional problems, those with anything from adult acne to premature wrinkles will go to a dermatologist. I reasoned that I could touch more lives for the better, and more immediately, as a dermatologist than I could in any other specialty. I became ardent about the powerful message I knew I had to offer. I chose to specialize in dermatology because I could see that I had the greatest effect on my patients' overall health when I could physically show the difference in their skin. In helping their skin look better, I also helped them become healthier in so many more ways. I am able to treat people of all ages, both men and women, and the breadth and depth of the fund of knowledge a dermatologist needs are an exciting challenge.

Consequently, I immersed myself in my education, knowing that my health and life depended on it. I got more than I could have dreamed of getting. I not only helped myself but I became passionate about wanting to help others on their own paths of growth and understanding. The vision was so obvious I wondered how it took me so long to get it. But often it is the things that are the most obvious that are the hardest to see. I had always wanted to be a doctor, but I finally felt the surge of self-confidence and determination I needed in order to reach my goal. As I began to live a life of purpose, I lost my extra weight without any conscious effort. It was as if it literally fell off my body. Not incidentally, my once-sallow skin quickly began to glow as a reflection of my newfound well-being. I felt a deep sense of joy and satisfaction in the work I was doing and the way I was able to affect others. My family and friends saw the changes in me and kept asking, "What are you doing?" It was as if I were changing right before their eyes, like magic. It wasn't magic at all. It was just my choosing to live—really live. My personal journey has given me great insight as I work with my patients. Then, too, because I am a working wife and mother dealing with many of the same challenges and issues as my patients, I can empathize with them on so many levels. I find that they feel comfortable confiding in me. After some sensitive questioning, I can get people to express concerns and problems that are having an impact on their health. "How did you know that?" my patients often ask. My answer: "I saw it on your face." And indeed, everything from sorrow to stomach ulcers can be detectable just by looking at the skin. By the same token, when patients come back to me a few weeks after starting my program, they have an un-mistakable freshness and vitality. I read that welcome message on their faces and in their skin as well.

On a personal note, when I run into people I haven't seen in a few years, including my colleagues in dermatology, they invariably do a double take and say something such as, "How do you manage to look younger and better every time I see you?" This, coming from other dermatologists, is one of the highest compliments I could ask for.

Now you can look forward to getting compliments, too. By fol-lowing my program, you'll have younger-looking skin no matter how old you are and no matter how much damage control you need. Each section of this book will take you through one step of my pro-gram. You'll be adding new behaviors and knowledge gradually as you go along. The reason I offer my program in four distinct steps is that most people become overwhelmed when trying to change too many behaviors and lifestyle patterns all at once. For example, you'd probably give up if I insisted that tomorrow morning you need to begin a daily skin-care regimen, modify your diet, limit your sun ex-posure, and start exercising regularly. But if you take your time, mov-ing at your own pace through each of my steps, you'll find that my program is both easy and effective. Success breeds success. When you achieve one goal and see the positive results in your skin, you'll be encouraged to go on to the next step. I speak from personal experi-ence and from helping scores of patients over the years. However, while I've arranged my steps in the order that works best for most people, feel free to skip around if you like. If your most important goal right now is to stop smoking, turn to my advice on page 81 and make this your step 1. Just don't be tempted to take on too many steps at once. Slow and steady wins the race, as the old adage goes.

I also want to underscore the fact that many of my patients never go on to step 4, which involves medical procedures such as Botox in-jections or laser treatments for blemishes. In other words, although I'm offering you the most up-to-date information on these modern miracles of dermatology in case you're a good candidate for them, I am proud to say that you may never need them if you follow the rest of my advice. Like many of my patients, you may be someone who not only can "forget the facelift" but someone who can forget the nonsurgical anti-aging treatments as well. And if you do opt for treatments at some point, you can be assured that you will get the most out of any procedures you and your doctor agree are appropriate for you.

Finally, interspersed throughout the book, you'll also see my "string of pearls." The pearls are words of wisdom that I use to motivate my patients. I like the idea of calling them pearls because their worth and patina are the result of the polishing that comes from coping with life's challenges in the same way that a pearl is the result of the oyster's solution for dealing with an intrusive grain of sand. The best part of my program, though, is how easy it is to follow. Just as I do with my patients, I'll guide you step by step while you learn to break skin-spoiling habits and begin to live the ageless skin lifestyle.

With this book, I am at last able to offer my program to you as well as to my patients. Turn the page and get on your way to ageless skin and vibrant good health. You'll see an enormous difference in your skin in a matter of weeks. If so much good can happen so quickly, imagine the difference a lifetime on my program can make. I am simply rolling out the red carpet for you and pointing you in a direction that is natural and easy. You can join my celebrity patients who not only look younger but feel younger as well, as birthday after birthday rolls around. Time and again in my practice I have seen proof that ageless skin translates into overall health and vigor so that every season of life can be a cause for celebration, discovery, and renewal. That happy outcome can be yours as well.

Your Skin Aging Score: Start Improving It Now!

1

Skin Basics

Not long ago while I was walking along Madison Avenue on my way home from the office, I spotted a friend I hadn't seen for several years coming toward me. She and I had been close when our children were preschoolers, but we had lost touch after the kids started elementary school. When I waved and caught her eye, she looked puzzled. Then as she got closer, her eyes widened and she let out a gasp. "I didn't recognize you at first!" she said. "You look younger now than you did when the kids were little. What's your secret?"

Here's the answer that popped out of my mouth: "I know all the medical facts about the skin and its ability to rejuvenate itself." Then I had to laugh because I knew she expected me to say something about what creams I use or what treatments I might have tried. "But seriously," I continued, "I feel strongly that while a little knowledge may be a dangerous thing, a lot of knowledge is liberating and rejuvenating. Everything I do to turn back the clock for my own skin stems from my knowledge about the skin."

That's exactly why, in this chapter, I will let you in on some fascinating medical facts about your skin. I want you, too, to be rejuvenated by knowledge about your skin. I am a big believer in science and the science of creating beautiful skin. Still, I can understand that you might be so eager to start improving your skin that you'll be tempted to turn to other chapters first. That's fine. However, promise me that you'll come back here for "Skin 101" once you've satisfied your curiosity about the other topics in the book. Remember, my "secret" for ageless skin isn't any single product or any single lifestyle change or any single treatment. It's a comprehensive program that begins with knowledge about the skin, and therefore with an understanding of the components of the plan and why they're necessary.

SIX FACTS YOU MUST KNOW ABOUT YOUR SKIN

If the eyes have been described as a window to your soul, I am here and now dubbing the skin as the window to your health and happiness. Your skin, like your heart, liver, or pancreas, is a vital organ that plays several keys roles in maintaining and enhancing your overall health. You can't survive without it. That's why taking care of your skin is so essential, not just for your appearance but for the rejuvenating effects this can have in general.

1. Your Skin Has Aesthetic Value

That is, it has the potential to be beautiful. Let's face it, this is what we all want and why I wrote this book. My patients often hear me say, "All I really care about is your skin." What they inevitably learn is that in order to help them have the most beautiful skin, we have to delve so much deeper, as you, too, will soon learn. They also learn that it is so much easier and more doable, even fun, than they expected. The aesthetic value of the skin is most important for many people, and I use that to my advantage in guiding people toward better overall health. Your skin is a powerful, very honest reflection both of the health of the skin itself and how well you treat it, and of your physical and mental health. The goal of this book is to help you have healthy, glowing skin, which reflects a healthy and happy you underneath.

2. Your Skin Protects You from Physical, Chemical, and Biologic Assaults from the Outside World

Healthy, youthful-looking skin is not only a great asset to your appearance but it is also vital for peak performance in the skin's role as defender of your well-being. The deeper layer of the skin is called the dermis, and the layer of mostly fat that lies beneath it, the subcutaneous layer, absorb shock and help you keep from getting too cold. Your skin also has blood vessels that help oxygen and nutrition reach the upper layers of the skin; nerve endings that provide sensation; and collagen, hyaluronic acid, and elastic tissue called elastin that give your skin resilience. Another more superficial layer of your skin, the epidermis, makes a pigment called melanin that gives your skin its color and tries to limit the damaging effects of the sun's ultraviolet rays. (See page 7 for more on the layers of the skin.) Finally, your skin is a barrier that is designed to ward off bacterial, viral, fungal, and other infections that are a threat to your skin and your overall heath. Your skin uses its own first-rate, first-responder network of immune cells.

3. Your Skin Gives You the Sense of Touch Through the Myriad Nerve Endings All Over Your Body

In this role, your skin can give you great pleasure. Think of how happy and peaceful you feel when someone you love strokes your cheek or gives you a kiss or holds your hand or hugs you. You have your skin to thank for the mood-lifting, stress-reducing results of the pleasurable sensations of touch. On the other hand, your skin sends you warning signals in the form of pain. You recoil quickly if you accidentally touch a hot surface such as an iron because your skin lets you know right away about the danger of burning. The same goes for extreme cold or cuts or abrasions. Your skin is an ever-ready alert system to keep you out of harm's way. Touch is the first of the five senses to develop in a human embryo. The skin tells your brain about sensations both pleasurable and painful by transmitting messages along a pathway of nerve receptors. Touch has been shown to play a crucial role in physical and emotional health. Nervous and cutaneous (skin) tissues in fact share the same embryological origins, which is why stress can cause skin problems. This is proof that my program, with its judicious blend of Western medicine and stress-reducing techniques, is the path to truly healthy skin at any age.

4.   Your Skin Is a Living, Breathing Filter

That's why cleansing your skin with the right products is so important. The wrong products can upset the natural balance of your skin and can actually lead to premature aging. I'll tell you more about that in chapter 3. Your skin is a permeable tissue that continually allows essential exchanges with the outside world. The cells in your skin let in oxygen, water, and minerals and at the same time eliminate toxins via perspiration.

5.   Your Skin Regulates Your Body Temperature Through Blood Vessels and the Process of Sweating

The skin is in effect your body's thermostat. When you're out in cold weather, your skin triggers shivering so the blood vessels will contract and keep you as warm as possible. But if there's a heat wave, you'll sweat to increase the blood flow to the capillaries, which in turn increases sweating. This process cools you off as the water evaporates from your skin.

6.   Your Skin Synthesizes Vitamin D

Vitamin D is an important nutrient for the health and strength of your bones because it allows calcium to be metabolized. It is produced in the epidermis when your skin is exposed to the sun. However, you need very little time in the sun, ten to fifteen minutes a day, to create all the vitamin D you need. This is more than adequately achieved from incidental sun exposure such as walking from one place to another or driving in your car over the course of any given day. The notion that avoiding the harmful effects of excess sun exposure will result in a vitamin D deficiency is a myth, and a dangerous one at that. I'll tell you lots more about your skin and the sun in chapter 4.

THE LAYERS OF YOUR SKIN

Your skin is made up of two layers on top of a layer of fat that attaches your skin to muscle and bone.

Epidermis

This is the top layer, the one you can see. It doesn't have any blood vessels and gets much of its nourishment from the dermis. The epidermis itself is made up of multiple layers, starting with the top layer of dead, flattened skin cells that we slough of with exfoliators. The epidermis varies in thickness from about 0.3 mm on the eyelids to about 1.5 mm on the palms. The average thickness is about 0.4 mm. The bottom layer of the epidermis is mostly made up of the only layer of dividing skin cells called basal cells, and melanocytes, which are pigment-forming cells that give skin its color. As the basal cells travel upward, they flatten and are called squamous cells. These cells continue to flatten as they become more compact and go through yet another name change to that of corneocyte. Each part of the process has a specific important role in maintaining a balance in the skin moisture and in serving as a barrier against the environment. It takes about four weeks for each skin cell to make the transition from basal cell to corneocyte, and about another two weeks for the corneocyte to slough off. This process is not synchronized, or we would lose all our epidermis every six weeks or so. We get some sloughing of skin cells every day, and sometimes we have to help move this part of the process along in order to have healthy, smooth skin. The epidermis also contains cells called Langerhans cells, which are the skin's own personal immune system.

Dermis

The dermis, which is below the epidermis, has many important elements that support our very existence, and, more important, help keep us looking young and beautiful: The dermis is 15 to 40 times thicker than the epidermis. The dermis contains blood vessels; nerves and nerve endings; hair follicles; erector muscles, which make the hair stand on end (causing goose bumps); sweat glands; sebaceous glands, which produce an oil called sebum that lubricates the skin; and lymphatic tissue to carry infection-fighting cells. The dermis is made primarily of the proteins collagen and elastin, which give the skin its suppleness and elasticity, and hyaluronic acid, which holds water, giving the skin texture, resilience, and a youthful look. (See chapter 11 to learn the new techniques for bolstering your own hyaluronic acid.)

Subcutaneous Layer

This is the layer directly under the skin. It is not actually part of the skin, but I mention it here because it stores fat and therefore has an impact on how your skin looks. For example, if you gain weight, you're more likely to end up with jowls and a double chin. This layer contains blood vessels as well as fat that acts as insulation—and sometimes just makes us fat. The layer is only a fraction of an inch thick on your eyelids, but it can be several inches thick on your neck or your tummy or your hips. Also, the subcutaneous layer works in concert with the epidermis and the dermis to regulate body temperature, and it attaches your skin to muscle and bone.

THICK AND THIN SKIN

The skin on the soles of your feet and the palms of your hands is thick and does not have hair follicles. The rest of your skin is thinner, softer, and more resilient. The skin on your lips is very thin and sensitive. It does not contain hair follicles or sebaceous (oil) glands, which makes your lips especially prone to becoming dry.

INTRINSIC VS. EXTRINSIC AGING

Intrinsic aging is a process that happens to everyone. It's the inevitable process of aging that occurs as the years pass, just as with the rest of your body. The rate at which intrinsic aging happens is determined by the genes you inherited from your family tree. However, the good news is that this natural process has relatively little to do with what causes your skin to look old. All of us over time gradually lose some collagen and elastic tissue, important components that keep the skin plump and smooth. Some lucky souls are blessed with genes that slow down that loss. Still, even people who are programmed to lose collagen at a brisker rate won't show particularly dramatic effects unless the causes of extrinsic aging accelerate the process. Chapter 4, "Avoiding the Skin Saboteurs," will help you prevent extrinsic aging and even reverse the damage once it's been done. Extrinsic aging is the result of outside factors—what you do to your skin. It is the part of the aging process over which you have a lot of control. For example, 99 percent of wrinkles are caused by sun exposure. This process is accelerated if you smoke and even more accelerated if you drink excessive alcohol and have a poor diet.

HOW YOUR EMOTIONS ATTACK YOUR SKIN

Everyone has a story—or many stories—about stress, hardship, and loss. A hormone called cortisol floods your system when you're dealing with stress. When that happens, all of your organs, including your skin, can be adversely affected. A fascinating study done by Israeli scientists showed that rainbow trout that were fed a single meal containing cortisol displayed signs of accelerated aging in the skin for a full week after ingesting the stress hormone. The researchers concluded that their results demonstrated the role of cortisol in speeding up the aging process in the skin of fish challenged by stressors. While there is yet no empirical evidence to prove that human skin reacts in the same way, I see that proof every day in my office, and studies are

Pearl: On your road of life, it's you who paves your way. You can choose to pave it with joyous moments and laughter and smiles, or you can choose to pave it with misery and pain and doubt. It's your life. It's your road—you pave it.

being designed to measure these effects objectively. Prolonged stress makes people look older than their years. Of course, cortisol is a hormone that is essential for life, and we would not want to eliminate cortisol from our bodies entirely. Cortisol is necessary for getting us through what our bodies perceive as "threatening" situations, and there are natural cortisol rhythms that our bodies expect and require for normal daily functions. However, too much of it too often is analogous to pressing your foot hard on the accelerator. When you go really fast, you use up a lot more energy and go through the fuel more quickly. This acceleration may get you out of a "dangerous" situation, but you also wear out the parts more quickly if you do that on a regular basis.

What's important to understand is that you don't actually have to be in a dangerous situation in order to feel as though you are. The mind is very powerful in directing how we handle life situations and in how our bodies respond to nearly everything to which they are exposed. Over each of our lifetimes we build millions of memories— often overlapping and redundant in many different parts of our brain, immune system, and other organs—around everything that happens to us. These memories affect, for better or for worse, how we respond to situations that call up those memories. For example, let's say several years ago you were in an automobile accident that involved hitting a tree that was near a lilac bush in full bloom. You escaped without serious injuries, but you were traumatized by the event. Now, whenever you smell lilacs you relive the trauma and your cortisol level shoots up. You may not even be aware that the scent of lilacs triggers this reaction. The memory may be deep in your subconscious, but you're experiencing stress all the same and the result may show on your skin in the form of rashes such as hives, breakouts, or potential wrinkles caused by extreme expressions. However, you can learn to recognize and outsmart those negative memory triggers. The trick is to desensitize yourself by purposely exposing yourself to a trigger and then using the full power of the mind-body connection to deactivate the association. In other words, smell lilacs or a lilac fragrance on purpose and tell yourself that your stress reaction is not based on a real threat at all. Say to yourself, "I like the fragrance of lilacs." Eventually, you'll remain calm even when you smell lilacs unexpectedly. You will have conquered your stress trigger and your skin will thank you for it! You can even undo much of the damage to your skin that was already done.

My point about memories does not apply only to the mind. It applies to nearly every organ, especially your skin. I believe that we understand so little about this that we don't even discuss it, but that we are addressing it from the end results. We say reduce stress, eat more of certain foods, watch the glycemic index of what you eat. And that's fine. I don't want you to try to understand this concept on a molecular level; I just want you to know it exists and that what you do to and for yourself makes a huge difference in how your skin looks. The good news is that you do not have to go through years of psychotherapy to identify each of your memory triggers in order to modify them. You just have to create new memories by looking at things from a different angle, an angle that you choose. You have so many choices about how you react to a situation and the effect it has on you.

YOU GET NEW SKIN EVERY SINGLE DAY OF YOUR LIFE

Some of the cells of the outer layer of your skin, the epidermis, slough off about once a day. This is the conclusion of a process in which the cells move up from the bottom of the epidermis to the top approximately every four weeks and then take another two weeks before they are sloughed off. However, there are always cells ready to slough off every day. They are replaced by new "young" cells. That's why, no matter how old you are and no matter how much damage has already been done to your skin, you can have younger-looking

Pearl: Never compare yourself to anyone else. As you follow my program, go for "personal best" and be proud of every little change you see in the mirror.

skin in a very short time. When you follow my Ageless Skin-Care program, you'll be giving your constantly renewable skin a chance to regain a remarkably youthful appearance before you know it. To that end, the next chapter teaches you how to calculate your score on my Skin Aging Test and gives you quick-start techniques for improving your score right away.

2

My Quick-Start Ageless Skin Guide for Instant Results

How old is your skin right now? Your chronological age notwithstanding, your skin may seem to be older than the number of candles on your birthday cake would suggest. In medical parlance, this is the difference between your *extrinsic* skin age (how old your skin looks) and your *intrinsic* skin age (how old your skin really is). The good news is that you do have control over your extrinsic skin age. Beginning right now, we're going to subtract years from your appearance. With my quick-start tips, you'll look younger *without surgery* in just one week. The difference in your skin will have people saying, "You look younger than the last time I saw you!" When that happens to me, I say: "I'm forty-two, but I'm thirty-five in *girl years*." The comment always brings a smile, and women instinctively know what I mean. Like it or not in this society, men of a certain age can be considered distinguished and powerful by virtue of obvious signs of aging such as graying hair and a lined face. On the contrary, women who look old tend to be regarded with less respect because they're "over the hill." I'm convinced that's why ageless skin is more important to most women than it is to most men, and I also believe that's why women have traditionally lied about their age. Now, though, you won't have to lie. You'll be able to reveal your true chronological age with great pride because in "girl years" you'll appear to be much younger!

To begin, take the Skin Aging Test. The goal is to *lower* your score week by week. That's why you'll calculate your score again at the end of each step on my program. You'll be amazed at the extent to which you've rejuvenated your skin. And the best part is that you can do this with relatively little effort. I'm going to teach you how to take care of your skin both from the outside and from within. You may be surprised at how easily your skin can look better than it ever has, and at the positive effect this will have on the rest of your life.

THE SKIN AGING TEST

Study your face in the mirror. You can use a 3x magnifying mirror if you choose, but I don't recommend using anything higher than that. There's no sense obsessing over every minute pore and wrinkle with a 6x magnification. The rest of the world couldn't possibly see that much detail, nor should they—or you. Stressing over a highly magnified version of your skin is counterproductive to achieving the goal of a truly more beautiful you. In addition, make sure to look at yourself in as natural a light as possible.

For each Skin Aging Factor listed on the chart on page 17, give yourself a zero for None, one point for a Mild condition, two points for Moderate, and three points for Severe. Total the columns and then add the results for your final score.

Pearl: This book is meant to be life altering without requiring you to make drastic, sudden, or unpleasant changes in your way of life. The changes you make will be gradual, joyful, and easy.

What Your Score Means

0–10: Keep Up the Good Work!

Chances are that you were blessed with good genes. Yet it's also a sure bet that whether you are twenty or thirty or forty or beyond, you are good to your skin. You cleanse it and nourish it, you use adequate sun protection, you eat right and exercise, you drink lots of water, and you sleep soundly. Don't stop now! Use the advice in every chapter of this book to add to your repertoire of skin-saving techniques and make sure that you'll maintain and enhance your youthful look for years to come.

11–20: A Few Changes Will Make a Big Difference!

You probably look older than you'd like. However, if you make a few simple changes, starting with modifying your sun exposure and minimizing the damaging effects of the sun and other stressors on your skin, you'll look younger fast. Better yet, you'll stave off future wrinkles in the bargain. You don't have to give up outdoor activities such as skiing or going to the beach. You simply need to learn how to protect your skin while you're in the sun. Contrary to what you may have heard, you need only a few minutes a day of sun exposure in order to manufacture vitamin D. Anything beyond a few minutes in the sun will

Skin Aging Factor

Skin Aging Factor	None (0 points)	Mild (1 point)	Moderate (2 points)	Severe (3 points)
1. Sallow skin tone (lack of a "glow")	_____	_____	_____	_____
2. Puffiness and dark circles around the eyes	_____	_____	_____	_____
3. Rough texture	_____	_____	_____	_____
4. Lack of resilience (Skin doesn't bounce back when touched. It stays depressed.)	_____	_____	_____	_____
5. Adult acne/Rosacea	_____	_____	_____	_____
6. Wrinkles	_____	_____	_____	_____
7. Brown "liver spots," also called "age spots"	_____	_____	_____	_____
8. White spots (liver spots so advanced that pigment is lost)	_____	_____	_____	_____
9. Broken blood vessels (showing as red spots or blotches)	_____	_____	_____	_____
10. Enlarged pores and blackheads	_____	_____	_____	_____

Total = _____

cause damage unless you are protected. I will show you ways to continue your lifestyle with a few simple modifications and tricks that will give you the best of both worlds—fun in the sun and healthy skin. Feel free to turn immediately to sections of this book that deal directly with your Skin Aging Factors. I designed this book for you to follow either step by step or to skip back and forth between chapters on your own. While I do prefer to have my patients follow my program step by step, I've learned that in this age of the Internet, people like to navigate at will to find information they're seeking. So go ahead and read the parts that most pertain to you before you read the rest of the book!

21–30: It's Never Too Late to Look Younger!

You will see the most dramatic results of all! In fact, I get great excitement and satisfaction out of working with patients who start out with a high score on the Skin Aging Test. I suggest that you follow my program in sequence and to the letter. That way we'll tackle all of your Skin Aging Factors and really make a difference. Be sure to have a picture taken of yourself in daylight lighting before you start. You won't believe how much younger you'll end up looking in one month. The picture is important because as lines and the signs of aging are erased, you won't remember what is no longer there. You will only see the smaller and previously much less obvious signs that remain. It is amazing how selective our memory is. We think we will never forget a wrinkle in our skin. Yet when it is gone, we have no recollection of its previous existence. We simply see any defects that may remain. I want you to be able to look at that photograph and remind yourself how great the improvement is. We are looking for a global difference in your skin—a rejuvenated, resilient face that looks and feels younger and healthier. A corollary of that outcome is that your facial expressions will take on a relaxed, more youthful appearance. You'll also find yourself making direct eye contact with people rather than averting your eyes. The reason is obvious: You know you look good and you don't need to "hide" your face. All of these changes add up to project a vibrant, ageless new you.

INSTANT RENEWAL TECHNIQUES

Now for those one-week wonder techniques I promised you.

Make Faces in the Mirror and Then Teach Yourself to Get Rid of Unnecessarily Extreme Expressions

We tend to look at ourselves in the mirror when our faces are at rest. That does not give a true picture of how we look when we are in motion. We all have dynamic expressions, whether they are smiling, laughing, frowning, showing alarm, or sometimes an odd combination of these. Most of us make extreme expressions that over time engrave lines on our faces as we keep making the same expressions again and again over the years. Test yourself by thinking up scenarios that will elicit various emotions and then glance in the mirror to see how your face is reacting to the emotion. It may be hard to think of the emotion while looking in the mirror, so look away, think of something intense, and then look in the mirror to see your expression. Do you raise your eyebrows a lot, causing forehead wrinkles? Do you squint? Wrinkle up your nose? Pout? Purse your lips? In his book *Blink*, Malcolm Gladwell eloquently describes work done by researchers Silvan Tompkins and Paul Ekman, which showed the connection between facial expressions and our emotions. Just by creating an expression, we elicit the emotion associated with it. For example, if you smile you'll begin to feel happy, and if you frown you'll begin to feel sad. Actually, actors using the Stanislavsky method have known this for many years. You clearly don't want to be expressionless, but what happens over time is that our expressions can become more and more exaggerated and actually end up looking unnatural. For example, before I started practicing this technique myself, my husband could always tell when I was on the phone with someone I was delighted to hear from, or if someone called me with good news. He would look at me, see me with an overexaggerated grin from ear to ear, and point out that it was a good thing the person on the other end of the line couldn't see the funny face I was making. Other times, people would respond to me as if I were angry or overly concerned. I could not understand why until I did this exercise and saw how exaggerated my expressions were when I was showing concern. I actually looked angry or worried, when I was not feeling those emotions at all. I see this every day, all day, in my office. I have since learned to use my voice more effectively to communicate my meaning and not rely on my face to do all the work.

Even worse, I woke up one day and noticed small lines starting to form along my upper lip. This was unacceptable. I noticed that I had gotten into a habit of pursing my lips a little when I was listening to someone else talk. I also see this every day, all day, in my office. I have since learned that I do not need to use my entire face to show that I am listening or that I care. I have trained myself to use my voice and my body language more effectively to communicate my meaning. I no longer make extreme expressions, so many of the lines have faded out.

You, too, can minimize a lot of wrinkles just by getting rid of extreme expressions. You'll look better immediately. The goal is to help you have more natural expressions that are more in tune with the message you are trying to convey. And over time as your skin cells slough off and are replaced by new ones, you'll actually have fewer frown lines and laugh lines. Do you remember your mother warning you not to make faces because you'll "freeze like that"? There's some truth to that old wives' tale. The more you "make a face," the more you end up etching that expression on your face. The skin at the base of the wrinkle that is now created is less resilient than the skin at the top of the wrinkle. This makes the wrinkle deeper and more pronounced over time. In fact, one effect of treatments such as Botox is that they "train" you not to tug against the relaxed muscles. That keeps you from making the extreme expressions that caused the wrinkles in the first place. In fact, if you do opt to have Botox treatments (see page 237), this exercise is especially important. You'll achieve and maintain the best results if you know how to minimize your expressions.

"Read" Your Face to See Whether Stress Has Affected Your Appearance

There's an old saying that "it shows on your face." That is often true. I'll never forget one patient I'll call Ellen Mason.* She arrived for a Botox injection on a crisp September morning, the kind of day that is imbued with the invigorating scent of autumn. Yet my trained eye told me that the fine weather had failed to affect Ellen for the better. Her brows were knit in a scowl and her skin had the telltale sallowness of a person who hasn't been sleeping well or getting much exercise. I also observed that her lips were often tensely pursed, causing feathery creases to appear around her mouth.

I asked her a few questions to help her feel at ease and to get a better sense of what I could do for her in terms of treatments to maximize her results. Before long she confessed, with several pained expressions, that she was scheduled to meet with her estranged husband and their lawyers later in the week. "I want to look so good that he'll be sorry he ever dumped me for his trophy girlfriend," Ellen said.

I asked her if, given the fact that he had betrayed her, she wanted him back. Apparently, she had never thought of the situation in that way. She was not used to thinking of herself first. I could see the lightbulb going off in her mind with all the possibilities now open to her. "You're right!" she said. "I want to look good for me for the first time in a long time." I smiled and said, "Let yourself be open to creating a thrilling new chapter of your life. Now you're free to follow your own dreams."

Instantly, an astonishing change came over Ellen's face. Her eyes took on an appealing sparkle, tension melted away, and the furrow between her brows all but disappeared. She got it. She understood that out of a clearly difficult situation that was not of her choosing she had an opportunity to do things she would never have dreamed of doing if she were still married. She would go out more with her

*Names and other details have been changed throughout the book to protect privacy.

Pearl: Success is the best revenge.

friends, travel, read books she never used to have time for—and control the remote!

Just then, one of my assistants walked into the examining room to get a piece of equipment. "Wow!" she said. "That treatment sure made a difference!" But I hadn't even injected the Botox yet. The "treatment" was all about starting the process of releasing Ellen from her bitterness and fear of being on her own. When that happened, her senses of passion and purpose were reawakened. Her whole face naturally relaxed and allowed the potential for inner transformation to start to show immediately on Ellen's face. With time and work, the transformation could become permanent.

Ellen did still need the Botox injection between her brows to help her on her way to a rejuvenated appearance, but I knew that the effect of the Botox would last much longer because she wouldn't be fighting it with extreme negative expressions. I also knew she would really be able to enjoy and appreciate the difference the treatment would make. True, we can't entirely eliminate our wrinkles just by feeling good about ourselves. Still, I was certain the treatment would work much better because Ellen had less reason to scowl in the first place. Also, burgeoning feelings of confidence and joy can result in rejuvenating life changes that will have continuous positive effects on the skin for a lifetime. These changes come from deep within us, and they help our skin far more than we ever thought was possible.

Ellen has been back for more treatments since then and we talk about our first meeting and the impact it had on her. She comes in looking radiant with just the right amount of makeup and colorful clothes that enhance her looks. She tells me of the books she's read, the places she's been, and we talk about what is next. Needless to say, this is one case that makes me feel very good indeed about the work I do. And I'm happy to say that there are countless more.

BEGIN MY AGELESS SKIN-CARE REGIMEN WITH MY UNIQUE "COMPLIANCE COMPONENT"

After you've studied the regimen beginning on page 26, turn to page 24 for a look at Ellen Mason's Ageless Skin-care Regimen Compliance Journal. Use hers as a model for your own Compliance Journal. The regimen will soon become an ingrained habit and you won't even have to think about it. I developed this journaling technique because too many of my patients used to be what we doctors call "noncompliant." In other words, even though my patients knew what to do to keep their skin clear and young-looking, they were "too busy" or "too tired" to follow the routines faithfully every day. These people were often convinced that they were doing exactly what I advised, but once they started to keep a journal, they saw much greater improvement. When we reviewed their journals together, we realized that not until they started documenting their efforts did they realize how noncompliant they had been. Unfortunately, if you fall into bed two or three nights in a row without removing makeup or applying a moisturizer, or if you head out the door without sun protection, you're courting trouble. Here's how to make sure you get into good skin-care habits:

Keep a Compliance Journal

Keep your journal either on your computer or in a beautiful bound notebook—whichever is easiest and most fun for you. Don't worry. This won't prove to be difficult or time-consuming. Just put a short-

THE AGELESS SKIN-CARE REGIMEN
Ellen Mason's Compliance Journal / Week One

Week One	Monthly Mask	Weekly Scrub	A.M. Cleansing	A.M. Moisturizing	A.M. Sunscreen	P.M. Cleansing	P.M. Moisturizing	🙂 😐 ☹
Sunday	✓	✓	✓	✓	✓	✓	✓	🙂
Monday			✓	✓	✓			☹
Tuesday			✓	✓	✓	✓	✓	🙂
Wednesday			✓	✓	✓	✓	✓	🙂
Thursday			✓	✓	✓	✓	✓	🙂
Friday				✓	✓	*Emergency kit—out late*	*Emergency kit—out late*	😐
Saturday			✓	✓	✓	✓	✓	🙂

cut icon on your computer desktop so all you'll have to do is click to get to your journal. Or leave your notebook with a pen attached on your nightstand so you won't have to search for it when you need it. Then simply check off each part of the Ageless Skin-care Regimen as you complete it, and give yourself a smiley face for each day you do the whole routine. Before you know it, the regimen will be second nature and you won't be even a little bit tempted to skip anything.

Put Your Homemade Skin-care Products in Pretty Jars and Bottles out in Plain Sight

This will make your products serve as visual reminders to stick to your regimen. And if you keep them in decorative containers, you'll be more likely to leave them for all to see. If you hide your skin-care products in the medicine cabinet, you may forget to use them.

Keep Your Store-Bought Skin-care Products in Plain Sight as Well

Again, concealing your skin-care products behind medicine cabinet doors increases the chance that you'll neglect to follow your regimen. Keep them on a vanity or dresser top so that you constantly see them and remember to use them.

Pearl: Keep a small jar of moisturizer in your briefcase or purse and dab on extra dollops under your eyes several times a day to keep thin, sensitive skin from drying out.

Add Some Soul-Soothing Atmosphere to Your Skin-care Regimen

Play your favorite calming music or CDs of nature sounds while taking care of your skin. This will help you enjoy the process, and that in turn will enhance the effects of the regimen.

Make Some "Emergency Cloths"

Saturate soft washcloths with a combination of a nonrinse cleanser and a moisturizer and seal them in zipper-style plastic bags. Keep them in your purse and use them on long airplane flights or anytime you're truly too overwrought to do the whole nightly ritual, such as when the baby is sick and keeps you up or you had to work very late or stayed out late. These emergency cloths are meant to be used within a few days to a week. After that, toss any unused bags and make a fresh batch.

MY AGELESS SKIN-CARE REGIMEN

Now here's my ideal skin-care regimen. It involves cleansing, sun protection, moisturizing, exfoliating, and tightening with masks. I don't usually recommend toners, although many people believe that toners are a key part of good skin care. In all my years of training, there was never a lesson on the importance of a toner, or what a toner offers that the cleanser and creams don't. Toners were invented by skin-care companies at least partially as a response to people complaining of their skin feeling oily and as yet another product to promote to the buying public. If you're as busy as I think you are, you don't have to worry that you are missing something important if you choose to skip the toner. Some people really find that they like using toners, and they feel that they help. If this describes you, keep using your toner as part of your complete skin-care routine.

I believe that there are a few essential basics for skin care, along with the skin-enhancing diet I'll detail in chapter 8, that apply to everyone, with a few minor variations, as you will see. The idea that most people can be compartmentalized into clean, straightforward categories of oily skin or dry skin is a myth. We all have a variation of combination skin with more oil around the nose and forehead and drier areas on the cheeks. True, your skin tends to get drier or less oily with time, and you may have other issues such as sun damage or adult acne. You should choose skin-care products that are right for your needs, or learn to make you own. I'll teach you all about how to do that in chapter 3, "Face Savers." Even so, the overall basic routine for skin care changes very little. In other words, if the areas of your skin that are dry are very dry, you'll choose a rich moisturizer, whereas if your dry areas aren't particularly dry, you'll choose a light moisturizer. But either way, you won't skip the moisturizer! The products you use may be different from those that another person uses, but the process is the same for everyone. So here is what I want you to do, and how I want you to do it, without fail.

First Thing in the Morning

   Use a gentle cleanser or mild soap—that is, one with little or no added surfactants. Apply with circular motions of your hands. Rinse or wipe off with a washcloth wrung out in warm water. Pat dry with a clean towel. Natural soap is made from oils such as olive, palm, or coconut. The word soap comes from the process of soap-making called saponification. This process combines sodium hydroxide or lye, oils, and water, and has an alkaline pH of about 9 to 10. All soap is made with lye. Once the saponification is complete, the final product is soap and glycerin, without any residual lye. The oils help create lather and help the soap last longer. Depending on the type of oil used, the soap can be more or less creamy. Also, glycerin is a humectant commonly used in soaps. The more glycerin in the soap, the more relatively moisturizing the soap is. Sometimes color and fragrance are added to the soap to make it more appealing to the user. Ideally the scents in soaps should come only from the essential oils since fragrance and color add nothing to the actual cleansing process and serve only to increase the potential for irritation and allergic reactions. Syndets (short for synthetic detergents) were developed to have a pH between 5 and 7 (which is closer to the natural pH of the skin). They therefore remove fewer lipids, which makes them gentler. Most of the cleansers we use today are syndets. There is also a third category called combars. These are a combination of soap and syndet. Their pH is between 7 and 9. Most deodorant cleansers are combars.

∽   Apply a light moisturizer with an SPF of at least 15. SPF stands for sun protection factor. I'll tell you more about SPF in chapter 4. Use upward strokes on your neck and forehead, and outward strokes on your cheeks, the area around your eyes, and between your brows. Never pull or press hard and never pull down.

∽   Apply either a foundation with a sunscreen, or a sunscreen product specifically made for facial skin. This is an extra layer of protection over the moisturizer with SPF. Again, stroke gently upward and outward, not down. If you are prone to acne, look for products that say noncomedogenic or nonacnegenic on the label. These products are least likely to clog your pores and contribute to your breakouts. If areas of your skin tend to be especially dry, use creams rather than lotions, since these are more moisturizing. I use the cream on most of my face, but I don't put it on my forehead, since that area is oilier.

Before Bed

∽   Use your cleanser again just as you did in the morning. If you wear contact lenses, remove them before cleansing, and try to get the hang of taking each lens out directly from your eye rather than pulling the skin around your eye taut, unless otherwise instructed by your eye doctor. Repeated rubbing or pulling day after day is not good for the delicate, easily wrinkled skin in that area.

Pearl: In addition to your morning and evening cleansing and moisturizing, you should cleanse and moisturize after any exercise session that makes you break a sweat.

⌒ Apply a rich moisturizer designed for use on the face. Unless the oily areas of your face are very oily, you should use a creamier moisturizer at night than in the morning. Your skin loses more water while you sleep than while you're awake. You can skip moisturizing your nose since it is generally oily. Apply the moisturizer about half an hour before putting your face on the pillow. This gives the moisturizer time to be absorbed so it won't end up on your pillowcase. Also, invest in soft, high-thread-count pillowcases to baby your face while you sleep. Be sure to launder them weekly with a mild soap, not a harsh detergent.

Once or Twice a Week

⌒ Use an exfoliating scrub to speed the natural process in which the cells of the epidermis, the outer layer of your skin, slough off. Most exfoliators are too irritating to be used daily.

Once a Month

⌒ Use a firming mask to tighten pores and improve blood circulation to your skin. You can choose the first day of the month, or any day that is easy for you to remember. Also, if you use an electronic calendar, add this part of the regimen as a recurring appointment.

If you follow my Ageless Skin-care Regimen without fail, you'll notice improvement within one week. By then the outer layer of cells will be sloughing off and you'll be getting brand-new ones that will be responding to the cleansing and moisturizing. This transformation takes time, but you really can start to see the effects in as little as a week. And at the end of one month, you'll see an amazing change for the better.

Even so, as I said earlier, surface care is not enough. Young-looking skin comes from the changes you make on the inside as well. I call this process an "inner makeover." Remember Ellen Mason? For her, the stress from a troubling marriage was the underlying issue that was accelerating the aging of her skin. Obviously, we all have stress that is greater or lesser at various times in our lives, and I'm not being as simplistic as to say that you have to be stress-free and happy in order to have great skin. Stress is part of being an active member of society. It is not possible, nor is it probably desirable, to eliminate stress completely since even blessings like having children, job promotions, and getting married are also known to be very stressful. What I am saying is that you can learn to manage your stress.

I use the story of my own loss to prove this point. When I was fifteen, I lost my younger sister to cancer. We had shared a room, nearly

Pearl: When traveling, pack a couple of soft pillowcases in plastic bags and use them instead of scratchy, detergent-laden hotel cases.

everything we owned, and our hearts. We had always told each other that we had an invisible glue so that nothing could ever separate us. She was very healthy until it hit. Six months later, that was it. By the time she was diagnosed, it was already too late. There was no treatment or chemotherapy available that could make her better. I had no choice about what happened to her, but I had a choice about how I lived my life afterward. Over the next ten years I began an intense emotional, physical, and spiritual journey that greatly helped me realize that we are all in a sense alchemists who can make "gold" out of "dirt." I was able to take the most difficult experience of my life, one I still to this day feel as acutely painful as I did nearly thirty years ago when I first lived through it, and help it evolve into a form that had life and energy that had so much good within it. I chose to honor the person that my sister was by trying to be a better and more sensitive person myself in my family life and in my role as a physician. I would try to look at concerns and conditions from a patient's perspective in my practice, and to be a strong patient advocate. I also knew from my education, and from my own experience, that this had to be accomplished from both the outside and in, as the skin drapes, covers, or reveals so much about a person. I found my calling. I also chose to become a journalist so I could reach a larger number of people and educate others about issues that are important for health and well-being. I also wanted to share my belief that every day is wonderful and precious. In fact, every day is a new opportunity to live and love

Pearl: Strive for personal best. Just do all *you* can do—and be proud of yourself!

Pearl: Make something good out of
everything, even things that seem to
have no good in them at all.

and work hard and really be your best, since every day is really a whole lifetime.

That's why I'm going to teach you in chapter 5 the techniques I teach my patients like Ellen so that they can examine their lives and find ways to ease their inner tensions on a daily basis. You can, too! The difference will look great on your skin.

Now, keep reading in order to learn how to evaluate store-bought skin-care products and also about how to whip up rejuvenating creams, scrubs, masks, and moisturizers right in your own kitchen.

Pearl: Every day is a lifetime.
Make the most of it.

3

Face Savers

There are many excellent skin-care products on the market. The key to choosing the right store-bought products is to become an educated consumer, and I'm going to help you do just that. You'll be able to do some serious comparison shopping by reading labels carefully in order to choose products that are right for your skin—and your wallet! Remember, the best products are not always the most expensive.

In addition, I'm going to teach you how to create your own formulations using items that are probably already on your grocery list, such as fruits, oatmeal, honey, yogurt, and green tea. This way, you won't be subjecting your skin to the irritating fragrances, dyes, and preservatives found in many store-bought products. You'll also be saving money, and you'll be able to make only as much as you'll need for each week so that your homemade face savers will always be fresh and effective.

Pearl: Discipline is doing the right thing when
no one is looking. There is no such thing as
getting away with anything. Your skin and your
body will reflect pretty quickly, one way or
the other, how you treat them.

NATURAL VS.
SYNTHETIC INGREDIENTS

Nature is full of wonderful ingredients that, when properly combined, work to renew the beauty of the skin. However, I'm not
against many of the synthetic ingredients in today's products. I get
questions all the time from patients and beauty editors at magazines
about whether natural ingredients are better than synthetic ones. The
assumption is that all natural products are safer and more effective.
The reality is more complex. Research has shown that if you take an
ingredient from nature and synthesize the identical ingredient in the
lab, the effect on your body is the same no matter which product you
use. In fact, sometimes synthetic ingredients are "new and improved"
versions of what is found in nature, and they may have a stronger or
more desirable effect with less irritation.

Not only that, but many of the "natural" herbal remedies on
the market today have never been tested, and may give you disappointing, or sometimes even dangerous, results. Certain herbal remedies can be good and of course they have been around for centuries.
Still, there are two major concerns that need to be addressed before
you start taking an oral herbal product or using a topical herbal

treatment. The first is whether or not the herbal treatment may have an adverse interaction with any prescription or over-the-counter medications you are taking. Consult with your doctor and your pharmacist before ingesting or applying any herbal treatments. Second, keep in mind the fact that the Food and Drug Administration does not regulate the companies that make herbal products or check to be sure their products really do what they claim to do or contain adequate concentrations or equivalent concentrations from batch to batch of the ingredients to be effective. You can visit www.herbalsafety.utep.edu for more information about the safety of herbal preparations.

KNOW YOUR INGREDIENTS

Deciphering the labels on skin-care products is easy once you understand the terminology. The list of ingredients is usually found right on the container, but it may be on the packaging. Remember, every single thing you put on your skin penetrates to some extent depending on the purpose. For example, exfoliants only need to reach the top layers of skin cells in order to loosen them and help slough them off. You wouldn't want exfoliants to penetrate too deeply since that would be abrasive and irritating to the skin. Other ingredients need to go deeper in order to cleanse and moisturize your skin.

Active Ingredients

These are the substances that directly effect changes in your skin. A good skin-care product should contain at least one active ingredient. Most products contain only one or at most two active ingredients, since the FDA frowns on products with multiple active ingredients. Active ingredients can work as antioxidants, moisturizers, exfoliants, and treatments for photoaging (sun-damaged skin), rosacea, acne, and other skin concerns. Common active ingredients include:

Antioxidants

Almost all of us have had a little too much sun exposure at some time in our lives, or a burn to the skin from cooking, or a bruise on the arm or leg from walking into something. All these events damage the skin cells with inflammation. The skin eventually repairs itself, and often the signs of the damage disappear or are diminished. However, if you keep exposing the same sites to more damage, over time the skin will not be able to recover completely and you will see evidence of damage in the form of scarring, brown spots, broken blood vessels, wrinkles, or sagging skin. Much of what I teach is about controlling the damage to skin cells from so many different sources, both internal and external. Inflammation is one of the most significant destructive processes that occur in the skin and other organs of the body. It results from a variety of insults to the cells such as the ones mentioned above. The most common causes of inflammation in the skin are not only the result of exposure to such insults as ultraviolet radiation, infections (including acne), irritant reactions, allergic or other immune reactions, poor diet, trauma, and burns but are also ongoing due to normal cell processes as the cells die and are replaced with new ones. We also know that as the skin responds to either insults or to normal cell processes, the pathway of inflammation includes a specific cascade of events and the formation of free radicals. Physically, the changes are visible in the skin in the form of redness, swelling, itching, pain, wrinkles, loss of collagen, and the acceleration of the aging process. The free radicals that are formed as a result of the insult are a necessary outcome of the inflammatory process, but they are also toxic to the skin and must be contained and neutralized. Antioxidants are naturally occurring molecules that neutralize the free radicals. They do so by providing electrons to the free radicals to restore a stable environment, with the goal of eliminating or at least minimizing the inflammation. Antioxidants are most commonly found in fresh foods such as fruits, vegetables, and nuts. A rule of thumb is to eat a variety of colorful foods in order to obtain the different antioxidants your body needs, such as vitamins A, C, and E, essential fatty acids, and more. When antioxidants are formulated for use on the skin, even if they don't penetrate through to the deepest layers, they can help to stop or slow the process of oxidation caused by free radicals and keep the cell membranes more stable. The problem with some antioxidants is that they themselves are not stable, so as soon as they are exposed to oxygen or light, they break down. The trick is to create antioxidants that are stable, effective, and not irritating, and to include them in adequate concentrations to exert an effect. Reputable skin-care lines do contain stable antioxidants that are effective. Examples of antioxidants used in skin-care products are grape seed extract, green tea extract, and vitamins A, C, and E. In addition, alpha-lipoic acid, melatonin, yeast ferment, and certain marine extracts are other ingredients available in skin-care products that may be both direct and indirect antioxidants.

Emollients/Lubricants

Emollients hold water on the skin, making it smooth and soft. Examples of emollients are aloe and shea butter.

Humectants

Humectants attract water to the skin from the external environment—that is, the air. Examples are propylene glycol and hyaluronic acid. (Remember from chapter 1 that hyaluronic acid is a humectant found naturally in the skin, as well.) The acid does not penetrate or directly add hyaluronic acid to the deeper layers of the skin. It works to pull extra moisture from the environment to help keep your skin moist and resilient.

Surfactants

These are ingredients in cleansers and shampoos that make soap lather and glide more easily across the skin. They are often very irritating and can cause breakouts that mimic acne.

Vehicles

These ingredients are the delivery system for the active ingredients. Even the best active ingredients cannot function unless they are properly transported to the skin. While vehicles are technically considered to be inactive, they are nearly as important as the active ingredients since they drive the active ingredients into the skin and hold them there. Water is the vehicle in water-based products. Water is usually listed first on the label. In the same way, mineral oil or oil will be the first ingredient listed for an oil-based product. Determining whether the product is water or oil based will tell you a lot about how easily the product will spread on the surface of your skin, how well the active ingredients will penetrate your skin, and what type of "feel" the product will have on your skin. Each vehicle has its pros and cons. Different vehicles are good for different skin conditions. For example, skin that tends to be especially dry will need an oilier vehicle. Keep in mind that vehicles that are alcohol based can have an irritating effect on the skin because they allow the product to penetrate very quickly.

Gels

Gels are alcohol or water based. They have a soothing feel when you put them on your skin and they leave minimal residue because the vehicle typically evaporates off the skin quickly. Gels traditionally were based on alcohol, but those products were often too drying for most skin types. Technology has advanced so that many gels are now water based, which makes them great for getting active ingredients into the skin without being overly drying in the process. These are commonly used for products for oily skin types and for sports gels that contain sunscreen, since they do not tend to run into the eyes when people are physically active and sweating.

Ointments

Ointments are typically oil based. Because they have little or no water or other liquid to evaporate, they tend to feel sticky and greasy and are less pleasant to use. They are useful however because they are very effective at helping to deliver the active ingredients, as long as the active ingredients can separate from the oil. The occlusive, or blocking, nature of ointments provides a waterproof barrier over the surface of the skin that helps to keep the skin hydrated by preventing water loss from the skin. This hydration further enhances penetration of the active ingredient. That is why ointments are especially useful for skin that is dry and thick, like the skin on the palms of the hands and soles of the feet, or for people who have psoriasis or eczema and who have thicker active lesions. It is also used in some formulations for the face for those with severely dry skin. Since ointments have little or no water content in and of themselves, they penetrate better and are most effective when applied to well hydrated skin, so they should be applied right after soaking, bathing, or showering. However, avoid greasy formulations if you tend to break out. Instead, look for products that are labeled as noncomedogenic or non-acnegenic.

Creams

Creams are generally water based with the oil-soluble ingredients forcibly mixed with the water by adding an emulsifier. Besides water, they also contain ingredients such as propylene glycol, which evaporate off the skin. This makes creams more aesthetically pleasing since they feel less greasy than ointments.

Lotions

Lotions are in many ways similar to creams but they have more water. This means the vehicle is thinner, and that makes lotions potentially drying for people with very dry skin. I usually recommend that you use a cream during the winter, especially at night when there is increased water loss from the skin, and lotions or lighter formulations of creams during the warmer, more humid summer months. Most people need creams on their legs and body all year round since these areas have less oil production and need more help in maintaining adequate moisture. The consequence otherwise is skin that can look reddish, flaky, or ashy, and feels itchy and more sensitive.

Serums

Serums can be either oil or water based. They are a relatively new and increasingly popular type of skin-care product because they contain increased concentrations of ingredients such as antioxidants that can have an anti-aging effect. They are good for all skin types. However, they are not usually moisturizing and are therefore not meant to replace your moisturizer or other skin treatment.

Preservatives

These ingredients do exactly what the name says. They preserve the product and thus extend the shelf life. They achieve this by killing bacteria, yeast, and molds. Look for products with a very low concentration of preservatives. Preservatives, like fragrances, often cause allergic reactions. Also note that some antioxidants, such as certain types of vitamin E (tocopherol), are referred to as preservatives since they inhibit the degradation of the product, thereby increasing its shelf life.

Dyes

These are artificial colors added only to make the product prettier. Avoid colored products when possible. There is no sense putting anything on your skin that isn't going to benefit your skin and may in fact harm it. It is difficult to avoid these altogether, but if you see a product with a long list of dyes (usually weird names and numbers at the end of the ingredient list), then move on to another product, or use with caution. Consider doing a test on a patch of skin on the inside of your forearm for about two weeks before using the product on your face.

Fragrances

Fragrances, like dyes, are only in the products to make them more appealing. If you can tolerate the fragrance, then there is no problem. However, if your skin tends to be sensitive, look for products that are fragrance free. Be sure not to buy products that are labeled as "unscented." These usually contain ingredients to mask the scent, which may also irritate your skin. Some products have a lovely fragrance from essential oils, which may provide function in the skin as well as a pleasing scent.

UV Blockers

These are sunscreen ingredients. They can be minerals such as zinc or chemicals such as cinnamate. Products containing UV blockers need to be applied in adequate amounts, regardless of whether the product is intended only as a sunscreen or as a lotion or foundation that has UV blockers among the ingredients. The single most important thing you can do for your skin is to protect it against the damaging effect of the sun. The rule of thumb is that the amount of the product that is sufficient to cover the entire body is just about as much as would fill a shot glass. Obviously, you need less than that to protect only your face and neck when the rest of your body is covered by clothing. Also, remember that sunscreens need to be reapplied at least every two hours in order for you to benefit fully from them. Beyond sunscreens, you definitely want to look for products that offer sunscreen protection. An SPF (sun protection factor) of 15 is the minimum you need. That number blocks out about 95 percent of the sun's harmful UV rays. An SPF of 32 blocks out 97 percent of those rays, and an SPF of 64 blocks out 98 percent. Remember, though, that sunscreen can't block out all of the potentially damaging rays, even if you apply it according to directions, which few of us do. You can hurt your skin if you bake too long in the sun, even if you're

Pearl: Time to burn without sunscreen (minutes) X SPF = new time to burn (minutes) For example: You typically burn after 10 minutes in the sun, without sunscreen. If you use an SPF of 15, it will take you 10 X 15 times longer to burn, or 150 minutes (which is 2½ hours).

wearing a sunscreen with the highest SPF. In other words, use sunscreen but also limit your time in the sun. Try to wear a hat and to go out early in the morning and later in the day, avoiding too much sun exposure between the hours of 10 A.M. and 3 P.M.

Miscellaneous

In addition to the primary ingredients explained above, there are other additives that you might find listed in the ingredients labeling of your favorite skin-care products. Here is a list of these ingredients and the main functions these ingredients serve.

- *Caffeine* is an anti-irritant and may enhance the effect of sunscreens.
- *Essential oils* are soothing and can help heal the skin.
  - *Geranium oil* is one of my favorites. I recommend it after procedures to minimize bruising. More medical research is needed to better quantify the effects of these ingredients.
  - *Grape seed oil* has vitamins, minerals, and protein and is good for all skin types.
  - *Carrot oil* has beta-carotene.

- *Jojoba oil* has beta-carotene, vitamins, and minerals. Very good for dry skin.
- *Evening primrose oil* contains gamma-linolenic acid, vitamins, and minerals. Good for sun-damaged skin.
- *Tea tree oil* is antiseptic. It is commonly used in acne preparations and for wounds.

C~   *Witch hazel* is soothing and antiseptic.

Beware of buying products that don't have a complete list of all ingredients on the label. Listing ingredients is now required by law. The exception is that if a formula is patented or otherwise "secret," an application must be submitted to the FDA but the ingredients do not need to be listed on the label.

When the FDA labels a product as a drug, stronger claims can be made and the active ingredients must be listed separately, and the active ingredients must satisfy a list of requirements for safety and efficacy. Many companies walk a fine line in that they want to be able to make products that can make some claims, but they do not want to be categorized as drugs since they are then subject to increased watchfulness by the FDA. They also have to have different and more formal testing and wait for FDA approval. This is very expensive and can take years. Most cosmetic and skin-care companies are very careful to word their claims to fall short of putting them into the category of requiring FDA approval. Remember, if the FDA labels a product as a cosmetic, all the ingredients can be listed together often in descending order of concentration. That means that vehicles such as water and oil usually come first, but there is no indication of the differences among the types of ingredients. You have to figure out the distinct functions of the various ingredients listed. In some cases, no active ingredients are included at all. Sometimes the active ingredients are listed with their concentrations, but even this can be misleading. For example, the pH, or acidity, of your skin and of the product, and other values, may make one ingredient at a lower concentration more potent than the same ingredient under different conditions. The ingredients also need to be in a concentration and formulation that will allow them to reach their intended targets. Reputable skin-care products meet this test.

Colors and fragrance are usually listed last, regardless of concentration, and sometimes the UV blocking ingredients are listed separately just for clarification.

INGREDIENTS TO WATCH OUT FOR

I warn you to steer clear of skin-care products with exaggerated claims. They are usually very expensive and sold mostly through mail order or on the Internet by companies you have never heard of before. A general rule to go by is that a product should underpromise and overdeliver. If the promise on the label sounds better than a facelift, don't waste your money, or at least be very wary. Since these products are not considered to be drugs, there is very little regulation of them. As long as they word their claims carefully they can say a lot without really alleging very much. I see ads all the time that start with a question: "Better than Botox?" They are not saying theirs is outright. By asking it as a question, there is somehow an implication that this is possible. My patients come in asking me about it as if it were a statement of fact. They seem to miss the question mark at the end. If you choose to read it as a claim, that is up to you. I am amazed at how many people—often highly educated people—can be so easily misled. The data is usually anecdotal, with very little in the way of controlled scientific studies to back the claim. This does not necessarily mean that the product is good or bad or dangerous. It means you should be cautious before accepting the hype and consider saving your money for products that have a more solid foundation.

Finally, you should check ingredients to make sure that they are compatible with your skin. Keep a list of ingredients you know you are allergic to or are sensitive to and avoid them when making or purchasing products. If you think you are allergic to a product, an easy way to check is to put a small amount on your inner forearm. This area is

generally less sensitive than your face or hands and it is readily acces-
sible, unlike your back, where most allergy testing is done. If you do
not get a reaction, this does not guarantee that you are not allergic (although if you do get a reaction, it's more likely to be a true allergic reaction than just an irritation). You may need to repeat the test over a few
days, or see your allergist or dermatologist for more in-depth testing.

Sulfa-based Ingredients

There are many people who have discovered that they have sulfa allergies after taking antibiotics that contain sulfa. If you are in this category, then you should also avoid topical products that contain sulfa.
There are plenty of products available that do not contain sulfa. If
you know you are allergic, read the label of every product before
you buy to make sure it does not contain sulfa. If you don't know
whether or not you're allergic to sulfa, then you are probably not.

Sodium Lauryl Sulfate

This is a type of surfactant that can be extremely irritating to the
skin. It is the main ingredient that creates lather in a soap. It is difficult to avoid it completely, especially if you use soap. Some soaps add
moisturizer to combat the drying, irritating effects of SLS. Most
cleansers designed for the face use little or no SLS.

Cocamidopropyl Betaine

This is another type of surfactant that is commonly used in many
shampoos, gels, and soaps. It appears in more than 600 personal care
products, including products for newborns, young children, and
those with sensitive skin. Many of these products are specifically designed for sensitive skin because they are considered to be less irritating than other surfactants. Ironically, cocamidopropyl betaine was
named the American Contact Dermatitis Society's 2004 Allergen of

the Year. Those sensitive to this ingredient ususally get a rash on the eyelids, face, scalp, and neck. The rash usually clears when use of the offending product is discontinued. However, you may need to see your dermatologist if the rash does not resolve within a reasonable amount of time, which I consider to be one week to ten days.

Parabens

This is the most widely used family of preservatives in the world. It is commonly used in cosmetics, skin care products, medications, foods, toothpaste, and other products. Although it seems to be safe for the general population, studies and reviews are underway to evaluate a possible relationship between paraben exposure and breast cancer and/or male reproductive dysfunction.

Synthetic Colors

As I mentioned earlier, their only purpose is to make the product look better. I firmly believe that every ingredient in a skin-care product should have a purpose that benefits the skin. Making the product look better in the jar is not one of them. The large majority of skin-care products contain synthetic colors. But there are more and more product lines that do not use synthetic colors.

Collagen and Elastin

When collagen and elastin are applied to the skin, the molecules are simply too large to penetrate down to the dermis where the collagen sits. This means you can't apply collagen on top of your skin and expect it to sink in and function as collagen. Nor can you apply the proteins that make up collagen and think they will restructure as collagen in your skin and therefore directly increase the collagen or elastin in your skin. The only way to get these ingredients into the skin intact is to inject them. When used topically, they do, however, provide excellent moisturization for the skin and may help other ingredients penetrate the skin more effectively. This may be very useful in helping your skin maintain its elasticity. It may also protect the collagen stores you already have, as well as allowing for an environment within your skin that will promote increased production for collagen. Even so, any product that leads you to believe that topical collagen and elastin can actually penetrate the skin is making a false claim and should therefore be avoided, in my opinion.

DR. DAY'S FAVORITE
SKIN-CARE PRODUCTS

Now you're armed with the knowledge you need in order to avoid skin-care products that are not right for you and choose those that will enhance and rejuvenate your skin. There are many excellent products out there. I'd like to share with you my own list of top favorite products that promote ageless skin.

Albolene

This inexpensive cream cleanser has been around for generations, and it is great for more mature, exceedingly dry skin. It is fragrance-free and liquefies on the skin. Its basic ingredients are mineral oil, petrolatum, paraffin, ceresin, and beta-carotene.

Good Skin

I have been fortunate to have worked in product development for several different product lines over the years. I am very proud of a line I have helped to create and formulate called Good Skin. The line includes cleansers, toners, exfoliators, moisturizers, serums, SPF products, and tinted moisturizers and foundations. The products are based on the needs I saw in my patients, and my own needs for effective, affordable skin-care products. It is very easy to determine which product is right for you just by looking at the packaging. The products are color- and name-coordinated according to the condition of your skin, such as acne-prone, red/irritated, dull or aging, or severely dry. The ingredient list is clear, and it keeps skin care simple and complete. The formulations feel great on the skin and leave the skin soft and smooth, not greasy or sticky. There are also some products that are great for solving specific problems that may arise like the acne spot treatment swab. In addition, the line is offered at an affordable price.

La Mer

La Mer is very expensive, but I have seen wonderful results with this line that includes body serum, cleansing gel, cleansing lotions, face serum, mist, moisturizing lotion, and tonic. It has been on the market since 1965. It was first formulated by a rocket scientist (really!) who had suffered burns during an experiment. He made a lotion of herbs and marine plants that helped his skin heal. This became the basis for the products on the shelves today.

Olay Regenerist

This eye and face serum contains amino-peptides that help renew damaged skin. There is solid science behind these ingredients, and other skin-care companies are now creating formulations that include various peptides for their anti-aging effects.

Origins

This line of products contains organic natural ingredients and essential oils like those I recommend in recipes for homemade products. You can select among the products that work for your skin concerns. My favorites are the Ginger Essence and the Gloomaway products. Devotees swear by this line.

Pond's

Pond's cold cream is a tried and true product that has been around since 1846, when a chemist named Theron T. Pond used an extract from the witch hazel plant to heal wounds. The current line contains the old standbys—cold cream for cleansing and dry skin cream for moisturizing—as well as several new antiaging products.

Udderly Smooth Udder Cream

This very affordable cream, originally used to keep cows' udders soft and smooth, is also really great for dry, chapped lips and the thick skin of the hands and feet. There are lots of varieties that have been adapted into creams and lotions for human use with added aloe, and vitamins A and D, but you could also just get the original udder cream designed for cows. The product is available at most health-food stores.

THROW AWAY OUTDATED SKIN-CARE PRODUCTS

Now you are aware of what to look for when you head out to buy skin-care products. However, before you go shopping for new products, throw away any products that have passed any listed expiration date. If no date is listed, use the following guide:

- Mascara should be used or discarded within eight to ten months if you haven't used it up by then.
- Foundation and lipsticks can usually be kept for about one year.
- Sunscreens and other products containing UV blockers lose much of their effectiveness after a year.
- Cleansers, lotions, and creams are generally good for one to two years.
- Eye shadows and blushes are usually good for about two years.

Also, use your nose. If a product smells moldy or different than it did when you bought it, even if it has not passed the expiration date, be safe and throw it out. Don't take the chance of using ineffective, outdated, or contaminated products. Get rid of them. Give yourself a fresh start with new products, and buy them in small enough sizes so that if they're not right for you, you won't be losing a lot of money by throwing them out. Small sizes are also good because if you do like the product, you can use it up while it's still fresh.

HOMEMADE FACE SAVERS

Speaking of fresh, why not think about making your own "face savers" right in your kitchen? The process is fast, fun, and economical. You can also share the experience with your daughter, your mother, or your best friend. My thirteen-year-old daughter, Sabrina, and I have a wonderful time in the kitchen blending fragrant fruits and aromatic teas along with other fresh ingredients. We put on fun music (taking turns choosing what "fun" is) and we talk while we create. She's learning at an early age, as my mother and grandmother taught me, that you're never too young to take care of your skin. Sabrina is also learning that no matter how busy our lives become, we can always make time for soul-soothing moments that we share with those we love. As you know by now, my credo is that when you tend to your body and your spirit, you are tending to your skin as well.

Also, think about getting your husband, your boyfriend, or your son in on the act. Men these days are becoming far more aware of good health practices, and they can get as interested as women in rejuvenating their skin. Witness the surge in men's magazines with articles about health, fitness, and youthful good looks. If you get your guy interested in having a little fun with you by making batches of homemade face savers, you might just get him to read the rest of the book so that he can turn back the clock right along with you!

Before making any homemade face savers, be sure all kitchen surfaces are clean. Wipe counters with a disinfectant, rinse, and dry with a clean towel or a paper towel.

I've divided the recipes into these categories: Cleansers, Scrubs, Masks, and Moisturizers. Within each category are recipes especially suited to particular skin issues such as dry skin or acne. Look through the recipes and select the ones best for your concerns and then stock up on the ingredients. Most are available at your supermarket, and the rest, such as essential oils, can be readily found in health-food stores.

Here are the skin-enhancing benefits of some of the key ingredients in the recipes I've given:

- **Aloe vera:** emollient, healing, soothing, anesthetic
- **Avocado:** rich source of vitamin E, soothing, emollient
- **Banana:** soothing, nourishing
- **Carrot:** gently exfoliating, nourishing, antioxidant
- **Cocoa:** antioxidant and contains caffeine, a protection against skin cancer
- **Cucumber:** cooling, hydrating, astringent, brightening
- **Egg:** tightening
- **Geranium oil:** anti-inflammatory, astringent, styptic; available at health-food stores
- **Green tea:** antioxidant
- **Honey:** antibacterial, soothing
- **Milk and yogurt:** astringent, soothing, emollient
- **Oatmeal:** exfoliating, toning
- **Papaya:** exfoliating, contains digestive proteins
- **Witch hazel:** astringent

Cleansers

These will gently remove makeup and the accumulations of oils. They are every bit as effective as store-bought cleansers. If you choose to do so, you can use these homemade cleansers exclusively. However, you should also use commercial eye makeup remover if you wear mascara or eyeliner. After using any of these homemade cleansers, rinse with water prepared as follows: Fill a pitcher with water and add your choice of peeled, sliced cucumber or sliced lemon with rind. Let sit for two hours. Overnight in the refrigerator is even better. Allow to warm to room temperature before using. This water may also be used to rinse off store-bought products. Prepare new water every two weeks. Don't forget to moisturize after cleaning your face.

Emollient Yogurt-Avocado Cleanser

2 tablespoons yogurt
1 teaspoon dark organic honey
¼ ripe avocado, mashed

Mix yogurt and honey in a small bowl until smooth. Add the avocado and mix well. With your hands, apply to your face and neck with gentle circular strokes for about one minute. Rinse your face and neck with prepared water or lukewarm tap water, or wipe off with a warm, damp washcloth. Pat dry.

Antioxidant Carrot Cleanser

1 small carrot, cooked and mashed, cooled to room temperature
1 egg, beaten
2 tablespoons prepared chamomile tea, cooled to room
    temperature
1 teaspoon coarse brown sugar

Mix the carrot, egg, and tea in a small bowl until smooth. Add the brown sugar and mix well. Apply to your face and neck with gentle, circular strokes for about one minute. Rinse your face with prepared or lukewarm tap water or wipe off with a warm, damp washcloth. Pat dry.

Pumpkin Wash for Dry Skin

5 tablespoons canned mashed pumpkin
1 tablespoon flaxseed oil
1 teaspoon olive oil
1 tablespoon yogurt

Mix the pumpkin and oils in a small bowl until evenly mixed. Add the yogurt and mix well. Apply to your face and neck with gentle circular strokes for about one minute. Rinse your face and neck with prepared or lukewarm tap water or wipe off with a warm, damp washcloth. Pat dry.

Acne Cleanser

¼ cup witch hazel
1 tablespoon aloe vera gel
10 drops tea tree oil
3 drops lavender oil

Mix all of the ingredients in a small bowl until well blended. Soak a cotton ball in the cleanser until saturated. Apply to your whole face or dab over affected areas of your face and neck. Leave on for at least 5 to 10 minutes, then rinse with prepared water, or leave on if desired. Use 2 to 3 times a day as needed.

Face Scrubs

Scrubs are exfoliators and they should be used no more than once or twice a week, unless otherwise instructed by your physician. Before using a scrub, use a cleanser so that you are starting with a clean face. Avoid getting into eyes. Rinse face and neck with prepared water or with lukewarm tap water, or wipe off with a warm, damp washcloth.

Healing Oatmeal–Aloe Vera Scrub

Oatmeal is one of my favorite ingredients to use in a scrub. It has been used for centuries to cleanse and soften the skin. It is also gentle in abrading off the upper layers of skin cells. It is excellent for all skin types, including acne-prone and sensitive skin.

½ cup raw oatmeal, ground coarsely
¼ cup organic honey
1 teaspoon extra-virgin olive oil
1 teaspoon aloe vera gel
2 teaspoons cucumber water

Mix all the ingredients together in a small bowl briefly, for a grainy scrub. Mix longer for finer scrub. Apply to your face and neck with gentle circular strokes for about one minute. Rinse your face and neck with prepared or lukewarm tap water or wipe off with a warm, damp washcloth. Finish with a cold splash of tap water to tighten your pores. Pat dry.

Busy-Day Alternative
Add ¼ cup raw oatmeal and 2 teaspoons organic dark honey to your favorite cleanser to create a scrub. Follow steps outlined above.

Exfoliating Papaya-Honey Scrub
Good for all skin types.

¼ papaya with seeds, mashed
2 tablespoons organic dark honey

2 teaspoons whole milk or whole-milk yogurt

3 drops geranium or rosemary oil

Mash all of the ingredients together in a small bowl. Apply to your face and neck with gentle circular strokes for about three to five minutes. Rinse your face and neck with prepared or lukewarm tap water or wipe off with a warm, damp washcloth. Finish with a splash of cool prepared water. Pat dry.

BUSY-DAY ALTERNATIVE

Start with your favorite milky cleanser. Add ¼ ripe papaya with seeds and 3 drops geranium or rosemary oil. Follow the steps outlined above.

Moisture-Rich Exfoliating Salt Body Scrub

Good for dry skin.

½ cup sea salt

¼ cup ground, uncooked oatmeal

6 tablespoons flaxseed oil

1 tablespoon extra-virgin olive oil

8 drops geranium oil

Mix all of the ingredients in a small bowl. Massage over your body and feet in the bath or shower for 3 to 5 minutes. Finish with a cool rinse. Pat dry.

Broccoli Face Scrub

Good for all skin types.

3 tablespoons whole-milk yogurt
1 teaspoon honey
2 drops rosemary oil
Florets of 1 stalk raw broccoli, cut into small pieces

Mix the yogurt, honey, and oil in a small mixing bowl. Mix in the broccoli tips. Massage the mixture into the skin of your face and neck with gentle circular strokes for 1 to 3 minutes. Rinse thoroughly with prepared or lukewarm tap water. Finish with a splash of cool prepared water. Pat dry.

Oatmeal and Yogurt Face Scrub

Good for normal to oily skin.

2 teaspoons ground, uncooked oatmeal
¼ cup plain, whole-milk yogurt
1 teaspoon almond oil
½ banana, mashed

Mix the oatmeal, yogurt, and oil in a bowl and let sit until the oatmeal is soft. Add the banana and mix with your fingers until evenly blended. Apply to your face and neck with gentle circular strokes for about 2 to 3 minutes. Rinse your face and neck with prepared or lukewarm tap water or wipe off with a warm, damp washcloth. Finish with a splash of cool prepared water. Pat dry.

Rose-Almond Face Scrub

Good for oily skin.

1 teaspoon rosewater
1 teaspoon spring water
1 teaspoon almond flour or ½ teaspoon finely ground almonds

Mix the rosewater, spring water, and almond flour in a small mixing bowl. Apply to your face and neck with gentle circular strokes for about 3 to 5 minutes. Rinse your face and neck with warm water or wipe off with a warm, damp washcloth. Finish with a splash of cool lemon water. Pat dry.

Honey-Sugar Hydrating Scrub

Good for oily skin.

1 teaspoon organic honey (sweet-clover or Illinois buckwheat
    honey if you can find it)
½ teaspoon brown sugar
2 tablespoons spring water

Mix the honey and sugar well in a small mixing bowl. Mix in the water. Apply to your face and neck with gentle circular strokes for about 3 to 5 minutes. Rinse your face and neck with warm water, using your finger pads to rub scrub off your face and neck. Finish with a splash of cool cucumber water. Pat dry.

Masks

Rinse face and neck with water as prepared on page 52 or with lukewarm tap water, or wipe off with a warm, damp washcloth.

Cooling Cucumber-Carrot Mask
with Witch Hazel Rinse

Mask

Good for normal/combination skin.

½ cucumber, puréed
1 tablespoon plain, whole-milk yogurt
1 carrot, cooked and mashed
½ avocado, mashed
1 teaspoon aloe vera gel

Rinse

2 teaspoons witch hazel
1 cup warm water

To prepare the mask, mix all the ingredients together in a small mixing bowl. In a separate bowl, mix the witch hazel and water and set aside. Massage the mask into your face and neck. Leave on for 10 to 15 minutes. Rinse with the witch hazel and water rinse. Pat dry.

Basic Oatmeal Mask

Good for all skin types.

½ cup raw oatmeal, coarsely ground
¼ cup prepared cucumber water (page 52)

Gradually mix the oatmeal with enough water in a small mixing bowl to make a paste. Apply to your face and neck and allow to dry for 10 to 15 minutes. Rinse your face and neck with warm water or wipe off with a warm, damp washcloth. Finish with a splash of cool lemon water. Pat dry.

Banana Oatmeal Mask

Good for normal/combination skin.

½ banana, mashed
¼ cup raw oatmeal, coarsely ground
1 tablespoon honey
2 tablespoons sour cream

Mix all the ingredients in a small mixing bowl. Apply to face with gentle circular motions. Allow to sit for 2 to 5 minutes. Rinse your face and neck with prepared water or with lukewarm tap water, or wipe off with a warm, damp washcloth.

Antibacterial Banana-Honey Mask

Good for oily skin.

½ ripe banana, mashed
2 teaspoons brewer's yeast
1 teaspoon witch hazel
1 teaspoon tea tree oil
2 teaspoons organic honey
1 egg white

Mix together all of the ingredients in a small mixing bowl. Apply to your face and neck with gentle circular strokes. Leave on for 5 to 10 minutes. Rinse your face and neck with prepared or lukewarm tap water or wipe off with a warm, damp washcloth. Finish with a splash of cool prepared water. Pat dry.

Cornmeal Mask

Good for normal/combination skin.

2 tablespoons cornmeal
1 to 2 teaspoons cucumber water (page 52)

Mix the cornmeal with enough water in a small mixing bowl to make a thick paste. Apply to your face and neck with gentle circular strokes for about 3 to 5 minutes. Rinse your face and neck with prepared or lukewarm tap water or wipe off with a warm, damp washcloth. Finish with a splash of cool prepared water (see page 52). Pat dry.

Almond Acne Mask

1 teaspoon ground almonds
1 tablespoon honey
1 egg white
1 teaspoon tea tree oil

Mix all the ingredients together in a small mixing bowl until evenly mixed. Apply the mixture to your face and neck with gentle circular strokes and leave on for about 3 to 5 minutes. Rinse your face and neck with prepared or lukewarm tap water or wipe off with a warm, damp washcloth. Finish with a splash of cool prepared water. Pat dry.

Simple Avocado Mask

½ avocado, mashed
2 teaspoons cucumber water

Mix the avocado and cucumber water together in a small mixing bowl until evenly mixed. Apply to your face and neck with gentle circular strokes and leave on for about 5 to 10 minutes. Rinse your face and neck with prepared or lukewarm tap water or wipe off with a warm, damp washcloth. Finish with a splash of cool prepared water. Pat dry.

Yogurt-Honey Soothing Mask
Good for dry skin.

2 teaspoons honey
1 teaspoon fresh lemon juice
½ cup whole-milk yogurt
1 egg white, beaten

Mix the honey, lemon juice, and yogurt together in a small mixing bowl until evenly mixed. Stir in the egg white. Apply the mixture to your face and neck with gentle circular strokes and leave on for about 5 to 10 minutes. Rinse your face and neck with prepared or lukewarm tap water or wipe off with a warm, damp washcloth. Finish with a splash of cool prepared water. Pat dry.

Yummy Chocolate Mask
Good for all skin types.

Chocolate is becoming more and more popular in skin-care products as its benefits become clearer. It contains the antioxidants flavonols, as well as caffeine, which may help protect the skin from sun damage. Recent studies done in mice using lotions that contain caffeine show that it may be protective against skin cancer. Chocolate is also useful as a moisturizer, since it is rich in emollients, which help seal in the skin's own moisture. For chocolate that is used in skin-care products, cocoa butter, cocoa powder, or cocoa extract are mixed with other ingredients to make the desired product. It is better to use the actual chocolate than the extracts.

Factoid: Dark chocolate has four times as many antioxidants as green tea.

½ cup cocoa
4 tablespoons whole-milk yogurt
3 teaspoons ripe avocado, mashed
¼ cup dark organic honey
3 teaspoons raw oatmeal, coarsely ground
1 egg

Mix the ingredients together well in a small mixing bowl. Apply to your face and neck with gentle circular strokes and leave on for about 5 to 10 minutes. Rinse your face and neck thoroughly in shower with warm water using a washcloth to wipe off any remaining mask. Finish with a splash of cool water. Pat dry.

Moisturizers

For a lotion base, all you need is water, oil, and an emulsifier. An emulsifier is an ingredient such as lecithin that holds the water and oil together. Make small quantities, since you will not be adding any preservatives. Each batch should last no longer than one week. Discard any remaining moisturizer after one week.

For these recipes you will need the following equipment:

- Saucepan filled halfway with hot water
- Heat-resistant china or metal bowl
- Hand whisk or mixer

Basic Body Lotion

½ cup water, at room temperature
1 tablespoon lecithin granules
½ cup oil (I usually use olive, almond, macadamia nut, or grape seed)

Pour the water and lecithin granules into a heat-resistant china or metal bowl. Cover the bowl and place in a saucepan half filled with hot water. Allow the lecithin granules to melt in the water. When the lecithin is just melted, remove the bowl from saucepan and stir the mixture. Slowly add the oil to the mixture until well mixed. Cover and leave to cool to room temperature.

You can experiment from here by using different types of oils, adding essential oils, steeping beneficial herbs into your water before you add your oil, etc.

BUSY-DAY ALTERNATIVE
Take store-bought lotion that you have, add essential oils such as 2 to 3 drops geranium or lavender oil, and apply to body.

Winter Lotion for Dry Skin

Geranium oil is good for supporting balance and rejuvenating dry skin conditions and for wrinkled and matured skin. Myrrh is a gentle oil that is an excellent moisturizer.

½ cup distilled water
1 tablespoon lecithin granules
½ cup olive oil
6 to 8 drops geranium oil
2 to 4 drops myrrh oil
40,000 IU vitamin E oil (1 to 2 open capsules)

Pour the water and lecithin granules into a heat-resistant china or metal bowl. Cover the bowl and place in a saucepan half filled with hot water. (Alternatively, use a double boiler.) Allow the lecithin granules to melt in the water. When the lecithin is just melted, remove the bowl from the saucepan and stir the mixture. Slowly add the oil to the mixture and let it cool to room temperature. Blend all the ingredients in a mixing bowl using a mixer or hand whisk for one minute. Store in an airtight container or jar in the refrigerator or keep in a cool place. Shake well before use.

Tip: I leave the jar upside down when I store it so that when I go to use it, I turn it over and mix it in one step. Nothing like saving time whenever you can!

BUSY-DAY ALTERNATIVE
Add geranium oil and myrrh oil to your store-bought vitamin E moisturizer.

Deep Moisture Skin Cream

1 tablespoon cocoa butter
1 tablespoon lanolin*
1 tablespoon coconut oil
1 tablespoon wheat germ oil
1 tablespoon spring water
1 to 2 drops almond oil

In a double boiler, or a metal or heat-resistant china bowl inside a saucepan filled with water, slowly melt the cocoa butter, lanolin, and coconut and wheat germ oils. Be careful not to allow to boil. Remove from heat. Add the water and almond oil. Occasionally stir while the mixture cools. Place in a clean jar and use over the next one to two weeks.

Green Tea Lotion

1 tablespoon soya lecithin granules
1 cup prepared green tea (leave 2 green tea bags or tea leaves soaking in hot water for a few hours to concentrate the tea as much as possible)
3 tablespoons green tea oil

Pour the green tea and lecithin granules into a heat-resistant china or metal bowl. Cover the bowl and place in a saucepan half filled with hot water. Put this saucepan over low heat to melt the lecithin granules in the green tea. Do not allow the mixture to boil. When the lecithin is just melted, remove the bowl from the saucepan and

*Available at any health food store

stir the mixture. Slowly add the oil to the mixture while stirring until well mixed. Cover and leave to cool to room temperature.

BUSY-DAY ALTERNATIVE
Add green tea oil to your favorite body cream or lotion.

Rose Lotion

1 tablespoon soya lecithin granules
1 cup rose water
⅓ cup cold-pressed sweet almond or safflower oil

Pour the rosewater and lecithin granules into the heat-resistant china or metal bowl. Cover the bowl and place in a saucepan half filled with hot water. (Alternatively, use a double boiler.) Heat over low heat to melt the lecithin granules in the rosewater. Do not allow the mixture to boil. When the lecithin is just melted, remove the bowl from the saucepan and stir the mixture. Slowly add the oils to the mixture while stirring until completely mixed. Cover and allow to cool to room temperature.

BUSY DAY ALTERNATIVE
Add ¼ cup rosewater to your favorite cream.

You are approaching the end of step 1 of my Ageless Skin-Care program. Your skin has no doubt already taken on a youthful radiance that has people commenting about how great you look. Better yet, when you follow my advice in the next chapter about how to avoid the six skin saboteurs, you'll be on your way to giving your skin every possible chance to repair existing damage and to keep extrinsic aging at bay from now on.

4

Avoiding the
Skin Saboteurs

I'm confident that by now your skin has already dramatically improved. That's a great feeling. Now let's use the momentum to tackle what I call the Skin Saboteurs. The reason I haven't asked you to confront these enemies of agelessness earlier in my program is that many of them are among the most intractable of habits. I have learned that when people have already begun to see positive changes in their skin because of consistent skin care with good products, they are far more motivated to make challenging lifestyle changes. Yet I want to stress that these changes are a must if you want to keep your skin looking young and healthy. The Skin Saboteurs can undo all the good gained from the Ageless Skin-care Regimen and from any treatments and procedures you may eventually choose to have done to enhance your skin. Fortunately, it's never too late to defeat the saboteurs and benefit from a lasting rejuvenating effect on your skin.

SABOTEUR NUMBER 1:
TOO MUCH SUN EXPOSURE

There is no greater adversary of ageless skin than overexposure to sun. You may have heard that getting too little sun will result in a vitamin D shortage and therefore lead to the risk of brittle bones or osteoporosis. That is a myth. True, sunlight helps your body create vitamin D, but you only need a very small amount of sun exposure and you get that by walking a few blocks or in the course of your normal daily activities.

Also, only the first step in vitamin D synthesis takes place in the skin with the help of exposure to ultraviolet (UV) light. The product, called cholecalciferol, or vitamin D3, is then sent first to the liver and then to the kidneys for further conversion to the final product called 1,25-dihydroxycholecalciferol. This is by far the most active form of vitamin D. It also means that if the kidneys are not working properly, vitamin D loses much of its effectiveness.

In addition, it is important to note that the vitamin D3 obtained from foods and supplements is identical to that created in the skin except for a few atoms that do not affect the vitamin's function. In other words, this means that ingesting vitamin D orally is much safer and just as effective as relying on skin-damaging sun exposure for vitamin D. If you take a multivitamin, make sure it contains vitamin D. Also, look for milk and other foods that are fortified with vitamin D3. In addition, foods such as margarine, eggs, chicken livers, salmon, sardines, herring, mackerel, swordfish, and fish oils (halibut and cod liver oils) all contain small amounts of vitamin D.

Far worse than any danger of a vitamin D shortage is the damage that sun exposure will do to your skin. A look at the parts of your skin that are almost always covered, such as your tummy or the area under your breasts, compared with the skin on your face and forearms is ample proof. You'll notice that the protected areas are much younger looking. You can even see a dramatic difference in the area of skin on your neck that is protected by your chin. You will see a patch of skin that is lighter and younger looking than the skin to either side of it. This part of your neck has its own built-in protection. And you were wondering why you need a chin! Now you know— to protect your neck from sun damage! This really helps to show how much a nice, very fashionable hat with at least a one- or two-inch rim can do to protect the rest of your face.

If you've purposely gotten a tan ever since you were a kid, probably with baby oil to speed up the process, the price you're paying now is thickened and wrinkled skin. Worse yet, cumulative sun exposure over years may also put you at risk for skin cancer, the most common form of cancer. Ultraviolet rays (composed of UVA and UVB rays), from the sun or from the tanning booth, are known to be complete carcinogens. This means that exposure to enough UV rays alone, without any additional toxins or cancer-causing agents, is all that is needed to cause skin cancer. The sun is also an immunosuppressant of the skin, which means that it can slow healing, and it leads to the breakdown of collagen. This process not only is the primary cause of wrinkles, which is bad enough, but it also slows wound healing and can make acne breakouts worse. Remember, too, that the sun's rays are dangerous even during the winter and on gray days. The ultraviolet

Pearl: Does your sun hat tend to leave a telltale crease on your forehead after you take the hat off? Attach a strip of moleskin inside the brim and you'll be crease-free!

rays that you would feel as heat are blocked by the clouds, but about 80 percent of the UV rays penetrate the clouds and reach your skin. More people get a sunburn after being out on a cloudy day than on a sunny day, when their perception of burn is increased because they feel heat from the infrared rays and take cover.

Still, even if you've been overexposing your skin to the sun, you can reverse a good amount of the damage if you change your habits now. As you've learned already, skin makes new cells every day and sloughs off the old ones. There are treatments you can do on your own or that your dermatologist can do for you to improve the health and look of your skin dramatically. But this must be part of a complete regimen, where you understand the need for sun protection, within reason, on a daily basis. I'll teach you sensible sun habits so your skin will look younger fast and stay that way. First, however, take this quiz, adapted with permission from the American Academy of Dermatology.

Skin Damage and Skin Cancer Risk Factor Quiz

1. If your hair is:
Blond or red, give yourself four points
Brunette, give yourself three points
Black, give yourself two points

2. If your eyes are:
Blue, green, or gray, give yourself four points
Hazel, give yourself three points
Brown or black, give yourself two points

3. If you have:
A lot of freckles, give yourself five points
Some freckles, give yourself three points
No freckles, give yourself two points

4. After one hour in the sun, if you:
Burn or blister, give yourself four points
Burn then tan, give yourself three points
Just tan, give yourself one point

5. Where do you work?
If you work outdoors, give yourself four points
If you work both outdoors and indoors, give yourself three points
If you work indoors, give yourself two points

6. If anyone in your family had skin cancer,
give yourself five points
If no one in your family had skin cancer, give yourself one
point

7. Where did you live before the age of eighteen?
If you lived in the South, give yourself four points
If you lived in the Midwest, give yourself three points
If you lived in the North, give yourself two points

Now, add up the points to see what your risk factor is. If you scored:

26–30 points, you are at very high risk
23–25 points, you are at high risk
16–22 points, your risk is average
12–15 points, your risk is below average

Protect Yourself Against Sun-Damaged Skin and Skin Cancer

Prevention and early detection of skin cancer are the keys to maximizing your chance for curative treatment. Prevention also means younger-looking skin rather than the leathery appearance of skin that has been overexposed to the sun.

Here are a few simple measures you can take to minimize your risk of skin cancer and prematurely aging skin:

Skin Cancer

There are three types of skin cancer:

Basal Cell Carcinoma is the most common and the most curable if caught early. Basal cell carcinoma typically looks like a pearly papule with little blood vessels and redness or even ulceration in the center. It also may appear as an open sore, a reddish patch, a pink growth, a shiny bump, or a scar-like area. It does not heal on its own and usually grows slowly. It occurs mostly on sun-exposed parts of the body and is most common among people thirty to forty years old or older who have had lots of sun exposure over the years.

Squamous Cell Carcinoma is the second most common skin cancer and in its precancerous state, it may simply appear as a flaky red patch. If left untreated, these cancer cells can eventually spread to distant tissues and organs. Squamous cell carcinoma usually occurs after years of sun exposure and mostly on sun-exposed parts of the body.

Malignant Melanoma is the least common form of skin cancer but the most deadly. The incidence of melanoma seems to be due mostly to genetic factors. However, some studies suggest that multiple sunburns, especially before the age of eighteen, may increase the incidence of melanoma. Melanoma most commonly looks like a brown to brownish black spot that can be flat or raised. Sometimes it can ulcerate and bleed. It occurs more commonly on sun-exposed parts of the body, but can occur anywhere including the scalp, palms, or soles, and even on the genitals, or in parts of the eyes.

For more information, contact the Skin Cancer Foundation, a respected international organization that is concerned exclusively with the world's most common malignancy—cancer of the skin. The mission of this nonprofit organization is to increase public and professional awareness of the prevention, detection, and treatment of skin cancer. The Skin Cancer Foundation achieves its mission through worldwide public and professional education programs aimed at increasing awareness about skin cancer, sun protection and safety, skin self-examination, children's education, melanoma understanding, and the importance of continuing medical education and international action. Whether you have experienced skin cancer or someone you know has, you will find extensive information about the different forms of skin cancer, treatment options, and physicians to help you on the foundation's Web site: www.skincancer.org. The Skin Cancer Foundation's Web site, as well as all of their educational materials, has been developed under rigorous medical standards and reviewed by leading experts in dermatology and in the treatment of cancer. In addition to the Web site skincancer.org, you can reach the Skin Cancer Foundation by calling 1-800-SKIN-490.

Minimize Your Exposure to the Sun Between 10 A.M. and 3 P.M.

The sun's most dangerous burning rays are ultraviolet B. These are called UVB for short. Think "B for burning." UVB rays are strongest

> *Pearl:* If you notice any change in a mole or beauty mark, have it evaluated by your dermatologist right away.

between the hours of 10 A.M. and 3 P.M. Make every effort to minimize your outdoor time during these hours. And remember, the closer you live to the equator, the stronger the sun's rays for more hours in the day, since there is more daylight time in these areas. The sun is also stronger at higher altitudes. In addition, snow, sand, and water reflect the sun's rays and greatly increase their intensity. If you ski or go to the beach, do everything you reasonably can to shield and protect yourself from the sun's rays. Of course, it is not a good idea to spend all your time indoors. The idea is to take reasonable measures to protect your skin from the damage the sun can cause, while still enjoying tennis, golf, walking, skiing, and all those other wonderful outdoor activities that are good for our health and well-being.

Don't Get a Tan, from Either the Sun or Tanning Booths

Tanning booths are not safe. I repeat—they are not safe. Numerous studies have shown an increase in the risk of skin cancer in young people who use tanning booths, and down the road these people will have premature wrinkles and thickening of the skin. A tan is the body's defense against the sun. To get a tan, the skin must be damaged. There is no such thing as a healthy tan. A tan is always a sign of sun damage. Did I drive this point home yet? Tanning used to be considered a sign of good health. It is now known to be quite the opposite for your skin. If you like the color of a tan, try one of the hundreds of sunless tanning products now available on the market. They come in all different formulations, from sprays to wipes, gel, lotions, and creams, and some add in exotic ingredients that enhance the feel and the quality of the color it conveys. (See "Sunless Tanning" on page 76.) These are the only safe ways to tan.

When your skin tans, it is a sign that your skin has been "hit." The rays of the sun penetrate to the layer of dividing skin cells and damage the DNA. Over time, enough damage leads to the changes we see: aging skin and skin cancer. Melanin production is revved up since these cells can absorb the rays of the sun with less damage. Think of these as the parasol that opens and shields the DNA of the dividing skin cells, at least to some degree, from damage. It is the mechanism that creates the tan that is the problem, not the tan itself. There is active, ongoing research to find a way to increase pigment production by ingesting a pill or through an injection in order to create a tan without causing damage. These treatments are still in the experimental phases, but they seem to offer the best hope for a true tan without sun exposure. People who tan more readily are therefore more naturally protected from sunburns and skin cancer, although they are certainly not immune. Skin cancer happens in all skin types. It also takes more time for some people to turn up the volume of pigment production. This is a genetically inherited trait, and these people are also more likely to have a sunburn— and the pain and damage that goes with it—before they tan. Some people don't even tan at all. They just turn red and then back to white. I see these people, grown people, all the time at the beach, lying and baking in the sun, red as lobsters. I always wonder what the fun is in it for them, since it must hurt and they don't end up with a tan, and they must already know this since they are now grown and have probably burned plenty in the past.

At the End of a Sunny Day
Be Sure to Moisturize

Sun exposure is very dehydrating for the skin. That's why people who have oily, acne-prone skin feel better. The sun makes the pim-

Sunless Tanning

At this point, you have not only begun my Ageless Skin-care Regimen, but you also have the ideal store-bought and homemade products to make the regimen effective. But remember, there is no cream or treatment that will reverse sun damage beyond a point. I see patients in my office every day who use all the most expensive products and want all the most expensive treatments but they keep coming in with a tan. In the winter, they go to a tanning salon to maintain the color they worked so hard to cultivate over the summer. Don't be like these people!

However, if you're a sun worshipper looking to reform, I do have some very exciting news for you. The current generation of sunless tanners work extremely well, unlike those streaky, orange versions we had years ago. Today's products come in every possible variety. There are sprays, wipes, gels, lotions, and creams. You can use the products yourself or have the very talented people trained in spas and salons apply them for you. These products all have the same active ingredient, dihydroxyacetone (DHA), but the manufacturers also add in a variety of other ingredients such as bronzers, shea butter, antioxidants, and more to make the product look and feel better on the skin. Remember, though, that tanners do not protect you against sunburn. You still need to wear sunscreen every day, all year round.

Rain or shine, cloudy or sunny, winter or summer, wear sunscreen without fail. Choose a product with a minimum sun protection factor (SPF) of 15. The SPF applies only to UVB protection, so make sure you choose a product that blocks not only UVB but also UVA. UVA rays are not as dangerous as UVB, but they still pose a risk. If you scored as a high risk on the quiz on page 71, choose an even higher SPF. In addition, check the label for ingredients. Zinc and titanium dioxide are the most effective physical sunscreens. If you're going to be outdoors for any length of time, particularly at the beach or on the ski slopes, apply your sunscreen generously, and reapply every two hours. Water, wind, sweat, and exposure to UV rays all cause sunscreens to lose their effectiveness. Incidentally, although beta-carotene and other vitamins have been credited in the press with being sun protective, they are actually not protective against UV rays to any significant extent and should not be counted on to prevent skin cancer or sunburn.

ples dry up because it dries the water out of the skin. This leaves the skin dehydrated, thereby making it temporarily less oily. Unfortunately, however, the sun also causes the sebaceous glands to enlarge, which in turn leads to enlarged pores and increased production of sebaceous oils, a known factor in the process that creates acne. Also, the sun is an immunosuppressant to the skin and can cause increased activity of *P. acnes,* the bacteria responsible for certain types of acne. In the long run, sun exposure causes you not only to get wrinkles but also to break out.

> *Pearl:* Chronic sun exposure causes your pores
> to enlarge because it causes the sebaceous glands,
> oil-producing glands in your skin, to increase in size.

Wear a Broad-brimmed Hat or a Visor or Carry a Parasol

Hats are pretty and stylish as well as protective, so get yourself a head-turning collection of hats for every season of the year to ward off the sun's rays. Visors work well, too, and they look great with sportier and more casual outfits. Visors are also less likely to give you "hat hair." Another option that won't ruin your hairstyle is to carry a parasol. The word comes from French, meaning "protecting from the sun," and chic women around the globe have been using parasols for centuries. I did a Google search and turned up plenty of inexpensive and romantic styles, from Japanese versions to pastel silk trimmed with lace. However, if visors and parasols aren't appealing to you, don't let worries about messing up your hair keep you from wearing hats. Find a hairstyle that isn't affected by hats and make a habit of slipping into the ladies' room to fix your hair when you get wherever you're going. Believe me, the protective effect of wearing hats far outweighs the problem of needing to run a comb through your hair a couple of extra times a day! And remember, for every extra inch of hat brim, you get a 10 percent lower risk of skin cancer.

Wear Sunglasses

Sunglasses not only protect your eyes, but they also keep the sun away from the delicate skin around your eyes and keep you from making extra wrinkles by squinting. Again, remember that the UVB rays are affecting you even on cloudy days and during the winter. Don't put away your sunglasses when summer's over! Wear them all year long. Also, don't forget that you have melanin in your eyes, so melanoma can occur there as well. If you have a family history of melanoma, be sure to get your eyes checked regularly and tell the ophthalmologist about your family history so he or she can pay special attention to any brown spots or irregularities and treat them appropriately.

Consider Wearing Sun-Protection Clothing

Particularly if you must spend a lot of time outdoors or if you're headed to the beach or the slopes for a vacation, look for special clothing with sun-protection factors built into them. This is a great investment for your good health, and a very smart anti-aging move. The clothes look exactly the same as regular clothing but they are made of fabric that has been treated so that it provides 30+ SPF UVB and UVA protection all day. By contrast, an ordinary summer shirt provides an estimated 5 to 9 SPF. That is dangerously below the minimum 15 SPF recommended by the American Academy of Dermatology. Sun-protection clothing is also designed to cover more of your body than the average short-sleeved shirt or tank top and shorts that many people wear during the summer. Check catalogs and Web sites that feature vacation- and beachwear for sun-protection clothing.

Check for Signs of Skin Cancer Once a Month

No matter what your skin type may be—that is, whether you burn in five minutes or never burn at all—spend a few minutes once a month to give yourself a thorough once-over to check for skin cancer. Do this in daylight lighting in front of a full-length mirror. It is a good idea to do your breast self-exam on the same day. If you see any changes in your existing moles or if you spot new moles or nonhealing growths, make an appointment with your dermatologist as soon as possible. Remember, although some people are at greater risk than others, everyone is at risk. One of the wonderful things about the skin is that it is on the outside, so we can see everything and skin cancers can be found early when they have the greatest chance of cure. A monthly self-check greatly increases your chances of finding any problems at an early stage. Precancerous and cancerous skin lesions can be safely and completely removed in your dermatologist's office. It is heartbreaking to see more and more young people, and people of every age, dying of melanoma when simple measures could be taken to minimize their risk and detect the cancer early when cure is so much more likely. One person dies of melanoma every hour in the United States. While the exact relationship between melanoma and UV radiation is unclear, it has been well established that the sun is damaging to the skin and can cause other types of skin cancer as well as the other signs of aging that we're working so hard to prevent and repair.

The bottom line here is that the single most important thing you do for your skin to keep it healthy and looking young and beautiful and resilient is to protect it from sun exposure.

SKIN SABOTEUR NUMBER 2: SMOKING

One of the reasons I chose dermatology as my specialty is that vanity is a powerful motivating factor when it comes to getting patients to take good care of themselves. I have a greater influence on my patients than their internists do, simply because I capitalize on my patients' desire to have beautiful skin. A prime example is my near 100-percent success rate in helping people to quit smoking, even though they've been ignoring dire health warnings for years. All I have to do is explain in detail how "smoker's squint" and the toxins in tobacco smoke cause crow's-feet, sunken cheeks, and a sallow complexion. Suddenly people start paying attention and asking for guidance in kicking the habit. As odd as this may sound, the specter

Pearl: Never point out what you think are your flaws. When someone compliments you on your young-looking skin, simply say, "Thank you." Of course, if someone asks you for your ageless skin secrets, share them gladly!

of premature wrinkles is a lot scarier to most people than the possibility of lung cancer or emphysema a couple of decades down the road!

I know, because I used to be a smoker myself. I started smoking on the sly as a teenager because I thought it was cool and that it would make me look older and fit in better with the popular crowd, or "BPs"—Beautiful People—as we used to call them. Well, as the years passed, my habit did indeed begin to make me look older! I was able to quit for a few months or years here and there without too much suffering, but something always got me back in. Even though I had already learned in medical school how damaging smoking was to my health in general, it was not until I specialized in dermatology that I learned the impact of smoking on the skin and specifically how it could speed up the aging process in my skin. One morning I took a long, hard look at myself in the mirror, and I had to admit that smoking was taking its toll on my looks. I made up my mind to quit, and I did it within a matter of weeks. I have never been an "antismoker" in that I never pass judgment on my patients. I am here to help and guide. I'm going to share with you, just as I do with my patients, my Fourteen-Day Countdown to Kicking the Habit, beginning on page 85. But first, just to entice you to think about being more motivated to kick the habit and allow your skin to begin rejuvenating, I'm going to give you the medical facts about how smoking affects your skin. Studies have estimated that people who smoke appear to be as much as ten or twenty years older than their nonsmoking counterparts by the time they reach midlife. Here's why:

1. Tobacco smoke, including secondhand smoke, dries out the surface of your skin. With repeated exposure, your skin will lose its resilience and elasticity at an alarming rate. A study of 123 nonsmokers, 160 current smokers, and 67 past smokers between the ages of twenty and sixty-nine led by dermatologist Jae Sook Koh, M.D., and published in the *International Journal of Dermatology* in 2002, found that premature wrinkles can appear in smokers as young as twenty. The overall results of the study showed that the risk of developing severe wrinkles was three times higher for smokers in all age groups. The same conclusion was reached by a study jointly conducted in the 1990s by the University of California, the Department of Veterans' Affairs, and the Kaiser Permanente Medical Group.

2. Smoking causes accelerated production of an enzyme (matrix metalloproteinase-1) that breaks down collagen in the skin. This means that you lose the youthful plumpness of your skin far more quickly than you would if you didn't smoke. By the way, sun exposure also increases production of this enzyme, so if you smoke while you're in the sun, you're getting a double dose of trouble.

3. "Smoker's squint" will etch crow's-feet in the delicate skin around your eyes as you repeatedly react when the smoke literally gets in your eyes.

4. Your nails and fingertips will turn yellow over time.

5. Feathery lines around your mouth will become more and more exaggerated as the years go by and you keep puckering up to puff on those cigarettes.

6. Particularly if you are thin, repeated sucking on cigarettes can cause your cheeks to look hollow and give you a gaunt, unhealthy appearance.

7. Smoking constricts your blood vessels so that the amount of blood carrying oxygen and vital nutrients to your skin is reduced, thus thwarting your skin's natural process of renewal. After every cigarette you smoke, your microvasculature—the pathways that blood follows in your system—needs at least five minutes to get back to normal. During that interval, you are literally suffocating your skin, and you do this many times a day!

8. Studies have shown that smokers are three times more likely than nonsmokers to develop psoriasis, a chronic, unsightly, and intensely itchy type of skin rash that can be controlled but not cured. It tends to be at least partially a genetically determined autoimmune condition, but smoking exacerbates it.

9. Nicotine has been shown to have a diuretic effect. This depletes the moisture in your skin and gives your skin a parched appearance.

10. A study of 1,000 people done by researchers at the Leiden University Medical Center in the Netherlands showed that smoking quadruples your risk of developing squamous cell carcinoma, a form of skin cancer. See page 72 for details on this disease. Though the disease won't make your skin look older, it could make you die younger!

These are all fine reasons to quit, but they are not the reasons you are going to quit. They are the benefits you will have after you quit. The reason you are going to quit is because you will want to quit. You will be convinced that it is your choice not to smoke, and that this concept of addiction in which you are held captive by cigarettes will simply not apply. Then the very good news is that when you do quit smoking, your body will almost immediately get to work repairing the damage. What a bonus! And over time, the effects of smoking will be almost eradicated, depending on how heavily you smoked. You can also speed up the process of skin renewal after you quit smoking by taking advantage of the advanced nonsurgical skin-rejuvenating treatments I describe in chapters 11 and 12.

Now, as promised, I'm going to teach you how to quit smoking once and for all in just fourteen days. If you start your countdown today, you'll be smoke free in just two weeks. Then in two more weeks, your system will be well into its amazing recovery process so that your skin will have already begun to lose the telltale signs of "smoker's face."

Dr. Day's Fourteen-Day Countdown to Kicking the Habit

Day 1: Start to tell yourself that you don't like to smoke. You don't even have to believe it. Just keep saying it. Then, as you are falling asleep that night and every night for the next two weeks, take a deep breath in and hold it for three seconds. Slowly breathe out and feel your whole body relax from head to toe. It should take you twice as long to breathe out as it took you to breathe in. Do this three times. As you feel yourself relax, feel yourself holding a cigarette as you usually do. Feel your hand and arm get heavier and heavier. Allow yourself to feel how annoying and uncomfortable it is to not have use of that hand.

Feel yourself walk away from the smoke and the heavy darkness within your chest, and walk through a curtain to clear blue skies. Push the curtain apart and walk right through. Feel the difference on the other side. Take a deep breath. Enjoy how good it feels, how light, how free. This is your choice. You are walking away from smoking. Your lungs feel light and clear. Your skin is glowing. Your energy level is up.

Day 2: Every time you see someone with a cigarette, say to yourself: "Thank God, that's not me." Don't look and say, "Oh, just one won't hurt." Say, "Thank God, that's not me." If you approach quitting from an angle that says this is all my choice, and no one is taking it away from me, then the process is so much easier. Quitting is liberating. It is not a punishment. When I first thought about quitting, I panicked. I thought, "What am I going to do without the cigarettes?" Well let me tell you, once I realized that it was my decision and I felt in control, I was able to throw my cigarettes away without hesitating, and I lost another ten pounds just from the increased energy and productivity I had from not having to stop what I was doing to find a way to go somewhere where I could have a one-minute cigarette in the freezing cold or rain.

Day 3: When your friend or colleague comes to get you to go out for a cigarette break, take a moment to reflect. What do you really have in common with this person? Is there more to it than the company of going out for cigarettes? You might be surprised at how many of the people you surround yourself with are just there to help you support your habit and how little you might have in common with them if you didn't smoke.

Tell them, "Not this time." Stay in and get some work done. You will feel better and once the moment passes, the urge will vanish. If you get busy you will forget about it and that will be one less cigarette for you. You are on your way.

Day 4: When you think about having a cigarette, just tell yourself, "I think I'll skip this one." This is not the same as quitting. It is just saying, "Not right now."

Day 5: If you've always used smoking to jump-start your brain when you need to do paperwork, chew gum instead. Research has actually shown that chewing gum increases your mental agility, and that chewing sugarless gum is good for your teeth. Do promise me, though, that you won't start chewing gum in public, especially if you're having a conversation.

Day 6: Calculate how much money you'll save in a year depending on how many packs a day you've been smoking. Then choose a treat you'll buy for yourself at the end of the year with the sum you saved by kicking the habit. Better yet, donate the money to cancer research or to any other cause that's dear to your heart. Get yourself really excited about what you can have and what you can do. Really count on those things so that not smoking becomes truly desirable. You are not losing something precious. You are gaining so much that is more important to you.

Day 7: Get your car interior cleaned and vow not to smoke in the car again.

Day 8: Get all of your clothes cleaned to get the cigarette smoke out of them.

Day 9: If you smoke with coffee, switch to green tea to break the association.

Day 10: If you smoke with a drink, fix a plate of crudités to munch on as an orally satisfying alternative. You'll also be getting some skin-friendly nutrition with lots of antioxidants and fiber!

Day 11: Get rid of all smoking paraphernalia, including ashtrays, cigarette holders, lighters, and cigarette cases.

Day 12: Get the cigarette smoke smell out of your home by having your curtains, drapes, carpets, and bedspreads cleaned.

Day 13: Have your teeth professionally cleaned and whitened.

Day 14: Swear to someone you love and would never let down (and who doesn't smoke) that you won't smoke without their permission. You can do this in your mind or you can actually tell the person. In my case, I silently promised my children when they were very little that I would never smoke again. As time went by, I never told them I had ever smoked, so obviously I couldn't ask their permission to smoke. This worked like a charm for me. Every time I thought I had an urge, I would think of them and say, "No way could I hurt myself when I have such loveliness to care for." I could never bring myself to betray my promise to my kids. The urge would pass very quickly and I would be so happy that I hadn't given in.

I only really ever even got the urge at parties when I had a drink and people were smoking. I am very happy to report that I can withstand that now as well without even being tempted. I know that promising someone you love that you'll quit for good will work for you, too. You'll have something to fall back on in a moment of weakness. You will not even dare ask. You will think about that person and forget about the cigarettes.

Now crumple up your last pack of cigarettes, throw it away, and never look back. You have done it. The cravings will come and go for the first week or so. Then the physical part is over. However, the mental cravings last much longer. You just have to work on your mental will to not smoke. Certain associations may trigger memories of smoking—the smell of coffee brewing in the morning, the clink of cocktail glasses when people are toasting, the sight of someone apparently enjoying a cigarette. Our memories, many of which are deep in our subconscious, influence how our bodies respond to a situation. But you have the power to override that response. That is why the first step I gave you regarding quitting is to keep repeating to yourself that you hate cigarettes and you hate to smoke. Eventually, that thought will pop into your mind and replace any desire to smoke that arises from memory triggers. And if at the same time you visualize yourself with beautiful skin, you will find that you will start behaving in a way that makes that vision a reality. You won't even want to reach for a cigarette any longer. And once you get to that point, nothing can stop you. It is all in our minds. It is what we choose. It is such a great choice to opt for beautiful, younger skin.

Pearl: When my daughter, Sabrina, was born I made up a mantra that I repeat to her—and now also to my son, Andrew—every night before bed:

Always remember to love yourself;
And believe in yourself;
And try your hardest to be your best;
Because you *are* the best;
And you can do anything;
All you have to do is try;
And you can do it.
I love you.

SKIN SABOTEUR NUMBER 3: EXCESS ALCOHOL

There's nothing wrong with enjoying a glass of wine with dinner or a drink with friends. In fact, drinking in moderation has even been shown to be good for your heart, particularly if you choose red wine. However, if you are in the habit of having more than one or two drinks a day, or if you binge-drink at parties or on weekends, you're not only endangering your health in general but you're making your skin old before its time. Alcohol dehydrates your skin, thus depriving it of the moisture that makes for a youthful glow. The dehydration also deprives your skin, and your body, of essential nutrients.

Pearl: Because excess alcohol dehydrates your system—and therefore your skin—drink spritzers at holiday parties where the fun will last for many hours. Try three parts seltzer and one part white wine. You'll be festive all night long without risking a parched-looking face the next morning.

In addition, alcohol dilates your blood vessels, a process that can cause your face to flush unattractively. True, this condition is usually temporary, but it can lead to the chronic red blotches characteristic of rosacea. (See "The Skin Saboteurs and Rosacea" on page 93.) Worse yet, excessive drinking can cause other manifestations of rosacea, such as unsightly broken blood vessels, and these are permanent unless you opt for laser treatments. (See chapter 12.)

Be kind to your skin as well as to your entire system by limiting yourself to one or at most two drinks a day if you're a woman, and two a day if you're a man. Remember a drink equals one 4-ounce glass of wine, one 12-ounce beer, or one shot of hard liquor. And if you do go over that limit, perhaps on a special occasion or a holiday, be sure to rehydrate your skin right away by drinking plenty of water.

SKIN SABOTEUR NUMBER 4: ALLERGENS AND IRRITANTS IN BEAUTY PRODUCTS

The majority of allergic reactions to beauty products are due to preservatives and fragrances. Almost any beauty product you use has the potential to irritate the skin on your face. This means that you should read the labels of hair gels and sprays, mousses, fragrances, shampoos, conditioners, body washes, and body lotions to be sure they don't contain any ingredients that you already know will trigger an allergic reaction in your skin. And if you aren't aware of any allergies you may have, but you find that you are breaking out or suffering from hives or dry patches on your skin, look to beauty products other than your skin-care products as the possible culprits. In particular, eliminate products that contain dyes and fragrances as much as possible. These ingredients add nothing to the efficacy of the product and are often the cause of skin conditions you'd rather avoid.

SKIN SABOTEUR NUMBER 5: SALT

If you have puffy bags under your eyes when you wake up in the morning, you are almost certainly consuming much more salt than you need. This is a problem not only for your skin but also, at least potentially, for your blood pressure. To eliminate excess salt from your diet, start by taking the salt shaker off your table. If you're used to adding a lot of salt to your food, some dishes may taste bland when you first stop doing that. However, your palate will adjust very quickly, and you'll soon find that you're enjoying the natural flavor of many foods you barely noticed before.

The second step in curtailing your salt intake is to limit your use of processed and packaged food when you cook. On average we consume about 6,000 mg or 1 teaspoon of salt every day. Guidelines suggest that those with high blood pressure or heart failure should have as little as 250 mg per day and that the upper limit for the average person should be 3,000 mg (about ½ teaspoon) or less. If you are very active or sweat a lot, you may need more salt than the average person. It is also known that women who eat foods high in salt prior to their menses may have increased headaches and other symptoms of premenstrual syndrome. With that in mind, take a trip through your supermarket and read the ingredients lists on the labels of canned soups and vegetables, crackers and cereals, bread, processed cheese, canned tuna fish and salmon, cake mixes, frozen dinners, and so on down the aisles. You'll be amazed at how quickly your intake of sodium could zoom far above what you really need. The solution is to rely mostly on fresh fruits and vegetables, fresh cuts of fish, poultry, and meat, and unprocessed cheeses. Then cook with herbs and spices instead of salt. See chapter 8 for plenty of recipes that will help you do just that. I have basically stopped adding salt to almost all of my recipes. No one has noticed yet in my house.

Finally, avoid fast-food establishments, which offer only heavily salted fare. In other restaurants, ask if your food can be prepared without salt. If the answer is no, go back to the menu and make another selection. When you wake up the next morning without unsightly bags under your eyes, you'll be glad you made a salt-free choice for dinner the evening before! If you do overdo the salt intake on any given day, it helps to flush it out by drinking more water. Initially, the salt will cause you to retain the water, but keep drinking and you will regain the balance. If you feel thirsty an hour or so after a high-salt meal, you are already behind on your water intake. Aim for adding three to four extra eight-ounce glasses of water to your daily total as an initial goal, and adjust up or down as needed. Just make sure you will be able to have access to a restroom, since you will need one more often.

SKIN SABOTEUR NUMBER 6:
EATING DISORDERS

If you suffer from anorexia or bulimia, you are wreaking havoc with your skin. Severely restricting your food intake, taking laxatives, and inducing vomiting all have profound adverse effects not only on your skin but also on your hair and nails. Of course, you are also damaging your health in general. If you suffer from an eating disorder, I strongly encourage you to seek counseling. Once again, I'm counting on the fact that you will be motivated to get help now that you know that you are causing your skin to look far older than it really is. I know that's not what you want, and I have faith that you'll decide to get your situation under control so that you can follow all of the advice in this book and have the glowing, youthful skin you deserve.

I want to congratulate you as you reach the end of step 1 of my Ageless Skin-Care program and embark on step 2, during which you'll add my unique Ageless Skin Inner Makeover in order to combat stress. In fact, stress is really Skin Saboteur Number 7. However, because stress involves a strong mind/body connection, I have set it apart from the other six Saboteurs and given it an entire step of its own in my

Pearl: There are some delicious salt-free or low-salt seasonings on your supermarket shelves with flavors such as garlic and herb, lemon and herbs, and spicy chili pepper. Use them and you'll never miss the salt!

The Skin Saboteurs and Rosacea

People who have rosacea should be especially careful to avoid or control the six Skin Saboteurs. If you are one of those people who blush easily or turn "beet red" when you are embarrassed, then you may be one of the millions of people prone to this condition. The exact cause of rosacea remains a mystery; however, anything that causes increased blood flow to the skin can lead to various manifestations of rosacea such as diffuse redness of the face, a rash that looks just like acne without the blackheads, broken blood vessels, and bulbous changes of the nose (more common in men).

Rosacea is generally treated by avoidance of factors that aggravate it, combined with a variety of over-the-counter and prescription oral medications and topical prescription medications. Sunscreen should always be used, every day, all year round.

Some of the most common factors that aggravate rosacea are:

- Sun exposure
- Alcohol
- Extremes in emotion
- Spicy foods
- Blushing
- Increased temperature, or extremes in temperature
  - Hot showers
  - Hot drinks

> - Going from cold outdoors to hot indoors with dry heat, or vice versa
>
> ⌒ Weather
>   - Wind
>   - Cold
>   - Humidity
> ⌒ Exercise

Ageless Skin–Care program. I find that my patients benefit greatly from this progression. I know that you will, too.

But first, take the time to recalculate your score on the Skin Aging Test that you first calculated on page 17, in chapter 2. I'm certain you'll find that your score has already improved significantly, which I'm sure you'll find thrilling, and I also know that you'll keep improving your score as you continue everything you learned in step 1, and go on to step 2.

The Ageless Skin Inner Makeover

5

Cleanse Your Spirit, Clear Up Your Skin

Emotional toxins are just as damaging to your skin as environmental toxins and bacteria. In chapter 2, you learned a three-part daily regimen for cleansing your skin, nourishing your skin with moisturizers, and protecting your skin with sunscreen. Now you're going to learn my three-part regimen for cleansing, nourishing, and protecting your spirit. I call the regimen "The Three Rs for Ageless Skin from Within." *Releases* cleanse your spirit. *Rewards* nourish your spirit. *Relaxation* protects your spirit. If you use the Three Rs faithfully and continue to follow my cleansing, enriching, and protecting regimen for your skin that you started in chapter 2, the combined effect will be powerful indeed.

I remember one patient, Ginger Wilson, a fortysomething woman who was planning her second wedding. A lifetime of imprudent sunbathing had bequeathed her with prematurely leathery and lined skin, but suddenly she had also developed a severe outbreak of acne not only on her face but also on her back. When she first came to me, here's what she said:

There ought to be a grace period between wrinkles and acne! Do they make turtleneck wedding gowns? Seriously, doctor, is there anything you can do? Every time I call the caterer or work on the seating chart for the reception, all I can think is that I'm going to look like a cross between my grandmother and my teenage daughter when I walk down the aisle. Help!

And help her I did, with the appropriate Western medicine and with my Three Rs for finding peace and serenity. I sensed that the challenge of planning the wedding was aggravating her acne breakouts in a major way. When I questioned her, this is what I learned:

I have three teenagers, and my fiancé has a teenage son and daughter. The kids are definitely not acting like a real-life version of the Brady Bunch! His kids and my kids end up arguing and saying mean stuff to each other every time we get together. They are all supposed to be in the wedding party, but I'm a nervous wreck about how that's going to play out. I just pray that they'll behave themselves and not spoil the big day. Of course, I also have all the usual wedding stuff to worry about, like my caterer never returns my phone calls, my DJ doesn't have any of the songs I want, and I almost died of sticker shock when I got the florist's quote. This wedding is supposed to be a dream come true, but it's turning into a nightmare!

No wonder my patient was pumping stress hormones at an alarming rate. Although I couldn't reduce the costs of throwing a wedding or broker peace between warring factions of the family, I could give her stress reduction techniques that she needed to begin immediately, along with the medications I prescribed for her acne and a chemical peel I recommended to improve the appearance of her skin and decrease some of the fine lines that were starting around her eyes and

Pearl: Fear is your only true obstacle in life. It begins in your mind and turns on your body.

mouth. I taught her the Three Rs and asked her to record her daily Releases, Rewards, and Relaxation in a Compliance Journal.

After you've studied my explanations of the Three Rs beginning on page 97, turn to page 101 for a peek at Ginger's Three Rs Compliance Journal. Use her examples as templates for your own journaling. I want you to record your entries every day while you're on my Ageless Skin-Care program. Make a promise to yourself that you'll do this! You'll be very glad you did. The Three Rs will almost certainly soon become second nature. That's the case for the majority of my patients. The Three Rs eventually turn into an emotional reflex, and you won't need to continue journaling them every day. However, life being what it is, situations will surely arise down the road in your personal or professional spheres that will cause an inordinate amount of stress. At those junctures, pick up your Three Rs

Pearl: When you're faced with a list of tasks, do the most difficult one first. The rest will seem like nothing after that—and you won't be worrying all along about how to handle the Big One!

Compliance Journal and begin recording your entries again to make sure that you don't let tension and anxiety wreak havoc with your skin—and with your health in general. Journaling your Three Rs is a tool that you can use for the rest of your life whenever stress—even "happy stress" such as starting a new job or moving to a new home—threatens to "show on your face."

Here are The Three Rs for Ageless Skin from Within:

RELEASES

Releases cleanse your spirit of any ill feelings you may be harboring—consciously or unconsciously—such as bitterness, self-pity, shame, and fear of going forward. Through your Releases, you will let go of constraints such as seeking the approval of others or blaming yourself for circumstances and events that are not your fault at all. One patient, Linda Michaels, was struggling with infertility. She came to me because she was experiencing the red patches typical of rosacea. I gave her a topical remedy for the condition, but I also probed gently during my intake interview until I found out about her worries over infertility. Here's what she told me:

> *I'm forty-two, and it looks like I waited too long to try to have a baby. Ronnie and I started trying right after we got married two years ago but every month I'd still get my period. I'd end up sobbing and I'd tell Ronnie that he should just divorce me and go find a younger woman. He's a year older than I am and neither one of us had been married before. He had told me how much he wanted kids, and now I was failing him. We had both been tested, and his sperm count was just fine. As for me, there was nothing actually wrong, like blocked fallopian tubes or fibroids or anything, but the doctors just said I had lowered fertility because of my age. It was bad enough being heartbroken myself, but the fact that Ronnie was being denied his chance to be a father because of me was totally devastating. Of course he would always reassure me that*

The Three Rs for Ageless Skin
from Within:
Ginger Wilson's Compliance Journal
Week One

RELEASES

Week One	Entry
Sunday	*I forgive myself for all those teenage summers in the sun with baby oil. Hey, I didn't know how bad it was for me! Now I'll do damage control for my skin and be happy about whatever changes I make.*
Monday	*I'm planning a wedding that pleases Brad and me—the color scheme, the menu, the music, the vows, everything. Right this minute, I'm going to let go of my need for approval from my family and his family about our choices. You can't please everybody, anyway, and trying to please them all is just making me walk around with a permanent scowl!*
Tuesday	*My fifteen-year-old daughter is driving me nuts. She's into body-piercing, and she says she won't take out any of the rings and studs for the wedding. She also has a tattoo on her arm. Okay, so be it. I am not a horrible mother. Jenny is just going through the usual teenage rebellion. I promise myself that I'll quit battling her on this issue—and quit pursing my lips every time I think about how she'll look in the wedding pictures.*

Wednesday	*I will stop beating myself up for getting into some credit card debt after my divorce. I'm not saying I couldn't have managed my finances better back then, and I'm not excusing myself just because I was rattled about suddenly being on my own. But what's done is done. All I can do is keep paying down the debt and make wiser moves from here on.*
Thursday	*I will find a beautiful dress that forgives me for weighing twelve pounds more than I did when I got married the first time. I'm not overweight according to my doctor, so I can accept how I am now. Brad thinks I'm sexy and that's what matters!*
Friday	*This just bubbled up from somewhere in my subconscious. When I was in the sixth grade, I shoplifted some makeup. I never got caught and I never did it again, but I felt horribly guilty. I now resolve to let go of that guilt that's been inside of me for so long.*
Saturday	*My son is dyslexic, and at the start of every school year I somehow think he'll "get better." Duh! Fortunately, David's tenth-grade English teacher is a gem. She already e-mailed me about the Resource Room for David. Okay, now I promise myself I'LL STOP BLAMING MYSELF for his disability. It's not because of something I ate when I was pregnant or anything! Breathe in, breathe out. Quit making those frown lines because that doesn't help and it just makes wrinkles!*

REWARDS

Week One	Entry
Sunday	I'm proud of myself because I took the time to do my first scrub and mask this morning.
Monday	I bought myself the new Sandra Brown novel in hardcover instead of waiting until it comes out in paperback.
Tuesday	I make great five-alarm chili!
Wednesday	I went on e-Bay and found exactly the candlesticks I've been wanting, and at a great price. I deserve them!
Thursday	I bought new foundation with sunscreen in it. A little expensive, but worth it! A great shade for me!
Friday	I got a French manicure.
Saturday	I feel good about myself because I had lunch with my aunt in the assisted-living facility. She was so glad to see me! And I brought a jar of my homemade blueberry preserves. She loved it!

RELAXATION

Week One	Entry
Sunday	Instead of reading the Sunday paper, I played badminton in the backyard with the kids. I'm going to wait until Monday to find out whatever bad news is in today's paper! I can't solve the world's problems this morning

so I might as well enjoy my family and all our blessings.

Monday   I shut the door to my office after lunch and told my assistant to hold my calls for fifteen minutes. Then I closed my eyes and pictured Brad and me on our honeymoon. We're going to Cancun. Ah! The stress from the morning's meeting with my boss just melted away.

Tuesday   I went to my weekly yoga class after work.

Wednesday   Brad and his kids were over for dinner, and afterward we all watched Comedy Central. Lots of laughs! Felt great! And his kids and my kids actually got along for once!

Thursday   The morning at work was totally stressful, so I didn't have the energy to relate to anybody at lunch. I ate at my desk with my headphones on and listened to Handel's "Water Music." Ahhh!

Friday   The kids are at their father's place for the weekend so I'm going to treat myself to a lavender aromatherapy bath. It's probably the most clichéd stress reliever in the world, but it works for me! Then I'll call Brad and see if he's in the mood for a candlelight dinner. Maybe after that we'll have a little, um, private time in the bedroom. ☺

Saturday   We all went to Mud in Your Eye and threw some pots. My worries moved to the back burner of my brain!

he had no intention of divorcing me and that he would love me even if we couldn't have kids, but I still felt absolutely awful. And our sex life turned into a creepy robot ritual because I was taking my temperature to see when I was ovulating and then it was like sex on demand. Awful! All the joy and spontaneity went out of it. Well, we finally decided to give up on the natural route and try in vitro fertilization. The whole procedure freaked me out. I had always pictured getting pregnant during a beautiful lovemaking session with the man of my destiny. Now I was in a sterile environment getting pumped with hormones while my husband was in another room—well, you know, "collecting" sperm. Ugh! I just shut my eyes tight and told myself it would all be over soon and I'd be pregnant at last. No such luck! We've tried three times already and I'm still not pregnant. I've pretty much lost all hope at this point.

After Linda told me all of that, I explained the Three Rs to her. Back home, Linda wrote a Release that freed her from guilt over her infertility, and she shared it with me when I saw her again. Here it is:

I will stop beating myself up for waiting until I was forty to start trying to conceive. I can't help it that I didn't meet the right man for me until I was thirty-eight and that he didn't propose until a year after that. From now on instead of replaying my regrets in my mind, I will focus on the possibility that I may someday get pregnant, and I will give some thought to whether I would ever want to adopt. I'll also give thanks for the new medical techniques that might help me overcome infertility. Most of all, I'll give thanks for my wonderful husband, and for the fact that he says he will always love me no matter what. I'm not a loser! I'm a very fortunate person!

I congratulated her on a beautiful Release, and I also encouraged her to look at the fertility treatments as an exciting adventure, shared with her husband, instead of as a grisly medical procedure. I suggested that she and her husband plan a romantic evening before their next appointment, toasting to their love with champagne and then enjoying physical intimacy for its own sake rather than thinking of intercourse only as a means to an end. And I recommended that on the day of the appointment, they should start with a leisurely brunch and pleasant conversation about anything *but* the impending procedure and the previous failures.

The result? Linda's rosacea subsided significantly and the overall appearance of her skin improved dramatically in a matter of weeks. Not only that, but the very next time she went for an in vitro fertilization, she conceived twins. She has since given birth to two healthy boys at the age of forty-three, and she continues to follow my Ageless Skin-Care program religiously. "No one ever mistakes me for my sons' grandmother," she told me with a smile. True, the pregnancy might have happened without the Releases. Yet what the Releases provided was a way for Linda to enjoy the process of trying to get pregnant and prepare herself to be at peace with whatever the outcome might be.

I began to use Releases myself when I was an overweight and unhappy high school and then college student plagued by the feeling that I was a disappointment to my parents and that I had somehow been responsible for my younger sister's fatal illness just at the time I was blossoming into a young woman. Irrational, yes, but I had always had the eerie feeling that as I became more attractive to boys, I was somehow leaching the life out of my pretty and popular sister whom I watched deteriorate day by day as she lay dying of non-Hodgkin's lymphoma.

I could see, on a deep level, far from my consciousness, that she was dying, but it was never discussed, and I never allowed myself to believe it was even possible. When I got a call to go to the hospital to say "good-bye," it came as a shock that reverberated within me for the next few years. Even after I went to see her at the hospital shortly after she died, I kept waiting for her to wake up. I could see the peace on her face, but I couldn't accept that she was gone.

When I left the hospital, I went to school and handed in a paper because I didn't want to get penalized for handing it in late. I behaved as if nothing had happened. I didn't tell anyone what had just happened, not even my closest friends. I didn't cry over my loss or let my feelings out for years after that day. My inability to express or understand my own deep pain and fear that this could also happen to me added to my feeling that my sister's illness and death were somehow my fault because of all those times I had been a little jealous of her popularity or of something she had that I wanted, or some other silly teenage sibling stuff that sisters grow out of and laugh about when they watch their own children grow. And I carried around a weighty sense of responsibility after I became my parents' only living daughter. I felt I had to make their dreams for me come true even if that had to happen at the expense of my own.

Only when I began keeping a daily journal of Releases did I find the peace and courage to be myself and like myself. I would write, for example:

I want to earn a master's in medical journalism, with a focus on science writing, and I'm going to do that even though my parents don't think it's a wise career path since I expressed interest in going to medical school. They are concerned I won't do both, even though I assured them I will. I release myself from needing their approval.

At least partly as a result of that Release, I was accepted into the program of my choice at New York University, where I was also given a position as graduate resident assistant, which gave me room and board as well as a stipend. I was able to live on my own. My goal was to write about medical issues and show that there are so many choices about health and well-being and that there are ways to die with dignity when the time comes. I wanted to understand more about why I lost my sister, who was also my best friend and soul buddy. I wanted to write about hospice care and about attending as a family to the person dying, and to those left to live without someone they love so much. I had felt very left out of the facts and psychology of my sister's illness.

My goal to write about medical issues including death and dying was realized when, during the time I was studying for my master's, I was lucky enough to get a job as a journalist for various medical magazines. I got to go to conferences and report on what was being said. A lot of these conferences were about cancer, especially a new type of cancer that affected the skin, being seen in people with a strange new immunodeficiency syndrome, now known all too well as AIDS. I had my first encounter with dermatology and I was intrigued. I would go on to write about this and other issues about cancer over the next few years. The money I made helped me stay independent and gave me confidence.

After that when I did go on to medical school, what I had learned at NYU, along with my own life experiences, informed my studies and made being a doctor have a deeper significance for me. And even though I had not purposely sought my parents' approval, I was thrilled that they were immensely proud of me. I had followed my own star, and I ended up pleasing them because I had set out to please myself.

Another Release I wrote in my journal was:

My sister's illness was never discussed openly in my family. As a teenager, I was left to make sense of it by myself and my conclusion was that I had caused her cancer. I am now letting go of that because I have learned during my studies that I was experiencing a phenomenon called "survivor's guilt." I am not at fault for her death. I can go on and live my life joyously and with the full use of my talents and desire to help others. I can appreciate, without guilt, that I had such a wonderful and beautiful sister, and I share with my children how special and beautiful she was.

Don't hold a grudge against yourself. We would forgive anyone else in a minute for the things we hold against ourselves for years. I hope that you will use Releases, as I did and as my patients do, to wash away the skin-spoiling effects of lingering self-destructive emotions. Look into your heart and mind and soul. Then rout out self-recrimination and self-blame. Let go of what you cannot change

> *Pearl:* Learn from your mistakes,
> forgive yourself, and move on.

from the past and stop replaying the past in your head. Your level of skin-damaging cortisol will drop and you'll see a remarkable difference in the resilience and texture of your skin in a very short time!

REWARDS

Rewards nourish your spirit, just as moisturizers nourish your skin. Rewards are daily acknowledgments of what you do right as well as what your gifts and strengths are, and they are also little treats you give yourself now and then, such as a pretty new shade of lipstick you've been wanting or a series of cooking classes at the local community college. People—women in particular—tend to put others' needs and desires ahead of their own and we sometimes forget entirely to indulge ourselves with soul-satisfying pleasures. The Rewards you'll learn to give yourself don't have to cost a great deal of money or require much time out of your busy life. Once you get into the habit of rewarding yourself, you'll find that you'll actually be better able to give of yourself to your family. As Cathy, a mother of three, said to me:

> *Before I started Rewards, I was always last on my own list. There were small things, like I'd take the poached egg with the broken yolk and give the perfect ones to everybody else. There were big things, like I was so*

Pearl: Each of us has different things to learn from everything around us and from every encounter we have with someone else—often in ways that are subtle and unintended by the messenger.

busy being Mom's Taxi for the kids' soccer games and scout activities that I never got together with my girlfriends anymore. And when it came to the budget, I barely bought any clothes for myself because I felt my husband needed to look good for work and the kids needed to look good for school. Without even realizing it, I was starting to feel deprived and angry. No wonder I was walking around with a perpetual frown! That was crazy because the whole thing was my doing, not my husband's or my kids'.

Cathy took my advice about giving herself Rewards, and to her amazement, she was able to allocate time and money for herself that she had previously imagined just wasn't available. Here's what she said:

I still take the broken egg yolk. But now I have a better sense of myself and I have allowed myself a life outside of my family. I'm taking computer courses with an eye to going back to work. I've also joined a book club where I've met some fascinating people, and I make a point of seeing my friends every couple of weeks for lunch. I also finally have some great-looking clothes, and I've been inspired to pare off a few pounds. And I've noticed in some recent photographs that my expression looks relaxed and content and that my fine lines are all but invisible. Of course, I've also been religious about my Ageless Skin-care Regimen.

My skin looks amazing in the mirror! And people tell me I look younger than I have in years. Looking so good is very energizing!

I have my patients Reward themselves every a day. I want you to do the same. The Rewards can either be positive statements about you, treats, or both. Remember, though, treats need to be good for your skin. Practice moderation, and try to think of some treats that have nothing to do with food or large purchases. There's no harm in an occasional ice cream cone on a summer day or a piece of chocolate cake on a special occasion, but don't overdo it. By the same token, don't go crazy with your credit card and then worry about how you'll pay the balance. Rewards should leave you feeling very good about yourself, not regretful or remorseful!

Many of my patients say they have trouble coming up with positive statements about themselves. The idea is to pat yourself on the back for even the smallest accomplishments or steps forward rather than chastising yourself for not being good enough or doing enough. For example, let's say that you have never used a weekly exfoliating scrub in your life. Now you've read about scrubs in the first chapter of this book, but you still haven't gotten around to using them. On your Ageless Skin-care Regimen chart, you don't get to put a check mark until you finally use a scrub. But Rewards are different! You can write something such as, "I bought this book about how to have ageless skin and I did my Skin Assessment Test. I'm proud of myself for taking a step toward caring for my skin and for my health in general." You'd be amazed how this self-praise will lift your confidence and motivate you to do even more. I can almost guarantee that before long you'll try a scrub and earn your Ageless Skin-care check mark. I know you'll be delighted with the results of your first scrub, and then you'll be able to write a Reward giving yourself credit for beginning to take good care of your skin. On the other hand, if you had hung your head and made yourself feel bad about reading the advice about scrubs but not putting it into action, I'll wager you'd have gotten stuck there on an emotional plateau and maybe even have stopped reading the book because you felt you'd never get around to making any changes for the better. So write your Rewards, no matter how tiny the increments may be toward one goal or another!

However, not all of your Rewards have to be goal-oriented. You can simply applaud yourself for something as simple as "I make really good spaghetti sauce" or something as meaningful as "I volunteer at the church soup kitchen because I care about people who are less fortunate than I am." All that matters is that the Rewards are a big hug from you to yourself. The beauty of this is that you don't have to wait for anybody else to give you approval! I sometimes actually envision myself as a little girl, and in my mind's eye, I wrap my arms around the child I once was, and who is still a part of my being, and give her a loving embrace. It makes me feel warm and secure and gives me energy and courage to rise to the particular challenge du jour. Recognizing that my need for this kind of positive reinforcement has not changed just because I'm all grown up is hugely uplifting for me. Try it! And whether you're writing your Rewards or giving your child self a hug, you'll be employing astonishingly powerful mood-altering techniques. The resulting uptake in your self-esteem plus your newly positive outlook will translate into better skin. People who stop focusing on what they *don't* like about themselves and start paying attention to what they *do* like get the inner radiance that shines out to the world through their skin.

Pearl: Within us we are every age that came before and all the experiences we have had. These are a part of us and a part of what makes our lives so rich and wonderful.

In the case of Ginger Wilson, my acne-riddled and weather-aged patient on the verge of her second wedding, Rewards helped her stop obsessing about the breakouts as she began to feel good about other, more significant aspects of herself such as her kindness and her marvelous sense of humor. She also started treating herself now and then to a little gift totally unrelated to the wedding. One of these was a hardcover book she wanted to read right away instead of waiting for the paperback. "I had been denying myself pleasures like that because I was worrying about wedding expenses," she confided. "But it felt so good to buy myself that book. Look, we'll pay for the wedding flowers whether I shell out $25.99 for a book or not! And reading the book takes my mind off the wedding for a while."

Before long, Ginger's acne attacks were fewer, farther between, and not as severe, and she barely picked at the pimples her skin was trying to clear. Also, her facial expressions were not as negative and extreme, so her wrinkles began to become less noticeable. In addition, she followed her Ageless Skin-care Regimen faithfully, sloughing off old cells and letting resilient new cells create a more youthful appearance. Only then did the oral and topical medications I had prescribed really kick in. That was because she was no longer punishing herself with worry about how she'd look on her wedding day and how she'd pay for everything. Also, I gave her a chemical peel to speed the process of cell renewal. What a difference! Yet neither the

Pearl: If you find yourself berating yourself in your head, make yourself end with a positive statement. For example, if you say to yourself, "That was so dumb!" add "But I still love me."

Rewards by themselves nor the oral isotretinoin and chemical peel alone, or Ginger's Ageless Skin-care Regimen by itself would have been as effective as all of them in concert. One of the hallmarks of my program is that stress-relieving techniques together with regular skin care plus pharmacological interventions exceed the sum of their parts.

I hope you'll start right away giving yourself daily Rewards. Again, have a look at Ginger's journal on page 101 for some inspiration!

RELAXATION

Relaxation protects your spirit in the same way that sunscreen protects your skin. Healthy forms of relaxation reduce stress, thus lowering the skin-damaging levels of cortisol. Unfortunately, a lot of people try to ease stress with unhealthy habits such as overeating, drinking too much, and smoking. While these attempts at coping with stress may provide temporary relief, in the long run all they cause is more misery, more remorse, and sallow, prematurely aging skin! In chapter 4, you found lots of helpful advice about how to drink in moderation or not at all and how to quit smoking. In chapter 7, you'll learn how to enjoy nutritious, skin-enhancing food without overindulging. For now, let's explore some of the many fun and effective ways you can relax your way to Ageless Skin.

Music, Music, Music

The seventeenth-century English playwright William Congreve, in *The Mourning Bride,* penned the often misquoted phrase "Music hath charms to soothe a savage breast." Yet whether you like his version or the popular one that refers to a "savage beast," the words are absolutely true. Agitated animals do indeed respond to the calming effect of music. Better still, just as a lullaby will send a child off to a sound and peaceful sleep, when *you* are in emotional turmoil, your "savage breast" will be soothed by rhythms and rhapsodies.

Classical music can be especially calming. I recommend volumes I and II of *The Most Relaxing Classical Album in the World—Ever!* The thirty-six selections on the double CD for volume I include such favorites as Johann Sebastian Bach's "Air on a G String," Samuel Barber's "Adagio for Strings," Pachelbel's "Canon," Claude Debussy's "Clair de Lune," and Edward Elgar's *Enigma Variations*. Volume II has eighteen selections, including Handel's "Water Music," Anton Dvořák's *New World* Symphony, Johannes Brahms's Waltz no. 15 in A Flat, and Frédéric Chopin's Nocturne no. 2 in E Flat. All of the selections are performed by top artists and orchestras.

However, popular music and folk music can also be good for your mental and emotional health, as long as you avoid songs with lyrics that are downers. Why not listen to some cheery foot-tapping tunes from Broadway shows? Among my favorites are the scores to *Guys and Dolls, Chicago,* and *Hairspray.* I also love all the new renditions of old ballads that have been recorded over the past few years by Rod Stewart, Michael Bublé, and others. My husband, born and raised in Iran, loves country music. I love that. There are some moving stories about life in many country songs. I guess he relates to it somehow. We also listen to a lot of Persian music. We even had a Persian band play at our wedding. I have always enjoyed Middle Eastern and Indian music, and I am so happy to see that my children like it as well.

In fact, music therapy is an accepted healing practice that has been acknowledged by Congress. Trained music therapists work not only with emotionally challenged people, but also with those who have neurological disorders such as Parkinson's and Alzheimer's. Music therapy has even helped reach children and adults who are locked in the isolation of autism. That's a powerful testimony to the "charms" Congreve so wisely wrote about so long ago. Go ahead and stock up your car with CDs. Get yourself a portable CD player or an MP3 player to use when you're walking or jogging. Play music softly in the background during meals, during lovemaking, and when you're indulging in a good soak in a bubble bath. Whether you've been fretting over an unexpected bill for a home repair or worrying about your aging parents or stewing over a mistake you made at work or smarting from the harsh words of someone you love, tension and anxiety will float away on wings of song. Your face will relax, frown lines will soften, and you'll lose the sallow skin tone that comes with negative emotions. The glow you'll see in the mirror will take years off your looks!

Enjoy the Soothing Sounds of Nature

Human-made music isn't the only source of aural stress relief. Think of how peaceful you feel when you hear such sounds of nature as birdsong, the rustling of leaves in a summer breeze, the gentle lapping of waves on the shore, the babbling of a brook, the rush of a waterfall, the cadenced patter of rain, the crunch of leaves underfoot on a fall day, the whisper of snow falling in a wintry landscape. Whenever you can, get away from the cacophony of ringing telephones, car horns, sirens, people shouting into their cell phones, and other sounds that assault your emotional well-being. Take a walk in the woods. Stroll along a beach in the moonlight. Or just seek some restorative solitude in your own backyard or garden. And when you can't actually go out into natural settings, simulate the effect by listening to commercial CDs of the sounds of nature. Then glance in the mirror and witness the skin-transforming effect that has taken place.

Take a "Mental Vacation"

A similar ploy involves closing your eyes for a few minutes and imagining that you are in a peaceful, safe setting. Call up memories of relaxing vacation spots you've visited or pleasant places from your childhood. "Listen" to the sounds associated with your private escape, recall in your mind's eye the beauty of your surroundings, and remember the special perfume of that time and place. You'll be instantly refreshed, and the result will show on your face.

On with the Dance!

Lord Byron, the famous English Romantic poet, wrote, "On with the dance! Let joy be unconfined!" Yet hundreds of years earlier, in about 700 B.C., the Greek poet Hesiod had already evoked the power of Terpsichore, the Greek goddess of dance, with these words: "For though man has sorrow and grief in his soul, at once he forgets his dark thoughts and remembers not his troubles. Such is the holy gift of Terpsichore." Even before that, dance had been a part of the social and religious life of humankind in cultures around the world at least as far back as prehistoric cave paintings like the ones in Central India and Australia, where the Aborigines live.

The lesson here is that dancing can most certainly elevate your mood, not only because of the rhythmic movements but also because the physical activity releases endorphins. These hormones are your personal inner antidepressants. As a plus, you'll also be listening to music so that you'll be getting the benefit of that proven relaxer at the same time. And it's worth noting that just as music therapy is a legitimate field, dance therapy today is helping countless people find their way out of emotional distress and impairment and move—literally—toward a serene way of life.

When I was studying for some of my bigger medical school exams, I would go to the gym or for a run, have some dinner, and then sit at my desk and study relentlessly for hours. However, I was wise enough to take "dance breaks" to get my energy level back up and clear my mind for more studying. I would put on my Rick Astley tape and dance my heart out. No one else was in the room, of course, and I would deny it if you ever told anyone. I put the music on loud so I could sing along as well. I sound so much better when the music is really loud.

Don't worry about whether you're good at dancing. Graceful isn't a requirement. If you're shy about this, play some music when you're alone the way I did when I was in medical school. Just let yourself move! Of course, you might also consider formal lessons in square dancing, ballroom dancing, or line dancing, especially if your boyfriend, husband, significant other, or child is interested in joining you. But whatever the case, you'll find that once you start dancing, you'll soon agree with the words of Bobby, the tap-happy lead in the Broadway musical *Crazy for You:* "I'm dancin', and I can't be bothered now!" That's just the feeling you need to evoke in order to ease the strained look on your face, get your blood to pump vital nutrients to your skin, and give your skin a youthful glow. Go for it!

Learn Yoga

Yoga devotees swear by the calming effect of this ancient practice. Consider taking some classes, preferably with a friend or your significant other so you'll be motivated not to skip any sessions. You'll get the overall benefits, plus benefits that will help your skin in particular. For example, the headstand prep involves putting the crown of your head on the floor and balancing with your feet off the ground and your knees braced against your elbows while your palms are flat on the floor to the side of your head. Practitioners say the headstand prep improves blood circulation, thus nourishing facial skin and hair as a result of stimulating what is called the "crown chakra."

Practice Meditation

Modern medicine has embraced the principles of mindfulness and meditation as true paths to relaxation and healing. These results, as you know by now, translate into ageless skin. I recommend reading *The Art of Happiness* by the Dalai Lama with Howard Cutler (Penguin Putnam, 1998) as well other books in this series.

Read a Book

I always take a book with me everywhere I go. This way if I have to sit around and wait, I'm never frustrated. In fact I look forward to these forced interludes because they give me time to read. Also, if I see one of my patients reading when I come in the room, we often spend the first few minutes talking about the book. If I have read it, we talk about our views. If I haven't read it, I try to get a sense of what the book is about and whether or not I would want to read it myself. We become a mini book club, and I find this is an ideal way to let the person get comfortable with me. Not only that, but her choice of reading material gives me an idea of who she is. Is she reading a mystery, a love story, a B novel, or one of the classics? It also helps me see her in her "natural" state. I get to see her facial expressions and that tells me so much about her skin and her chronological age, all of which helps guide my treatment recommendations. Even the way my patients talk about the books they read and the effect the books have on them is interesting to me.

Books have the power to transport you away from your own concerns and to engage your mind and spirit. All of that can help you relax. I can guarantee that if you sit tapping your foot in exasperation in a doctor's waiting room or in an airport when a flight is delayed, your face will contort in ways that are not good for your skin. But if you come prepared with a book and think of the waiting period as an unexpected gift of time for yourself, your expression will soften and your skin won't be subjected to wrinkle-forming grimaces.

Try Aromatherapy

Aromatherapy involves the use of certain essential oils to release scents that can, among many other results, produce a calm state of mind. Lavender in particular will soothe your soul and soften the tension lines on your face. Try a lavender aromatherapy bath, enhanced by candlelight, music, and perhaps an escapist novel to get you away from your worries.

Let There Be Light!

Seasonal affective disorder, or SAD, is a documented phenomenon that occurs because of a decrease in serotonin—our "happiness hormone"—during prolonged periods of gray skies and rain. Particularly if you live in an area where the weather isn't often sunny, such as the Pacific Northwest, consider investing in one of the sunlight-simulating lamps that will brighten not just your home but your mood as well. There is no risk of excessive UV exposure. These are not tanning lamps. So why walk around feeling blue and therefore etching gloomy expressions into your face when investing in a simple lamp can cheer you up and relax your face?

On the other hand, you can use mood lighting to soften the ambience of your home after a day spent in the glare of fluorescent office lights. Candles, already mentioned as a good accompaniment to an aromatherapy bath, can work magic at dinner. And room-light dimmers have a relaxing effect as well. Bonus: Your skin will look especially lovely by candlelight or in the gentle beams of a dimmer. Take advantage of that when you're enjoying intimate moments with the one you love.

Get Creative

An ongoing study of elderly adults by Gene D. Cohen of George Washington University, sponsored by the National Endowment for the Arts and the National Institute of Mental Health among other organizations, has shown that people involved in such pursuits as painting, jewelry making, and writing are happier and healthier than those who have no creative outlet. Cohen, the author of *The Creative Age: Awakening Human Potential in the Second Half of Life* (HarperCollins 2000), maintains that it's never too late to benefit from "creative fitness." You won't be surprised that my take on this is that anything you do that boosts your morale and your physical well-being will improve your score on the Skin Aging Test. So throw some pots, or try your hand at knitting, or take a course in writing poetry. Creativity doesn't have to result in huge artistic accomplishments that get public recognition. Anything you do that taps your inner urge to make something new will leave you feeling better—and therefore looking younger and better as well.

Laughter Really Is the Best Medicine

In biblical times, the wisdom that laughter is good for us was already apparent. Here's a quote from Proverbs 17:22: "A merry heart doeth good like medicine, but a broken spirit drieth bones." And by extension, a broken spirit "drieth" your skin as well! In fact, the Latin origin of the word "humor" means fluid or moisture.

I also love this quote from the eminent seventeenth-century physician Thomas Sydenham: "The arrival of a good clown exercises more beneficial influence upon the health of a town than of twenty asses laden with drugs." His long-ago assertion has been backed up recently with empirical medical research. Dr. William F. Fry, a psychiatrist and emeritus associate clinical professor in psychiatry at Stanford University, reported an absence of stimulation of the stress hormones called corticoids and catecholamines when people were engaged in laughter. Dr. Fry and his associates also showed that laughter boosts the immune system. All of these effects are good for your skin. Beyond that, your face looks much better when you're smiling than when you're scowling!

Reach Out to Others

Helping others is good for your health. A ten-year study conducted by scientists at the University of Michigan of 2,700 residents in Tecumseh, Michigan, reported that those who volunteered for community organizations had fewer colds, headaches, backaches, ulcers, asthma, and arthritis than those who didn't volunteer. The volunteers in the study also reported eating better and sleeping better after having begun their outreach work. Also, a study done at Harvard University showed that people who watched a film of Mother Teresa helping children in Calcutta experienced an increase in their immune system response. Similarly, in their book *The Healing Power of Doing Good* (Fawcett, 1992; iUniverse Paperback 2001), Allan Luks and Peggy Payne offered evidence of a "helper's high" that serves as a stress reliever. Now you know one more way to relax your frown and avoid ending up with a face that's engraved with the evidence of anxiety. We each give in our own ways. I volunteer one morning a week at the Bellevue Hospital dermatology clinic in New York City. I get the opportunity to supervise budding dermatologists as they treat patients with a wide variety of skin conditions. I find that besides the pleasure of having the opportunity to help the patients, who are less fortunate than most of us, I look forward to my Tuesday mornings because I somehow always learn more from the residents than I could possibly ever teach them.

Harness the Power of Touch

Research has proved that touch is as essential to your health and well-being as food and water. Babies who are deprived of touch literally waste away, a phenomenon that was first brought to light in 1915 by a pediatrician named Henry Chapin. He visited orphanages and found that infants, in spite of being well-fed, were dying because nobody was cuddling them. Later, neuropsychologist James W. Prescott studied three areas of the brain—the cerebellum, the prefrontal cortex, and the limbic system—to show how touch promotes well-being. Put this vital information to work for you whenever you can. Start by giving bear hugs to your friends and family members. Children in particular are great spontaneous huggers, and having small arms wrapped around you is a guaranteed upper. If there are no children

Pearl: Are there people in your life who put you down in order to build themselves up? Smile politely and be glad you're not as emotionally needy as they are!

in your life at the moment, why not borrow some? You could volunteer to be a Big Sister, or to read to children at the library, or you could give a neighbor or relative a respite from child care while you reap the benefits of an outing to the zoo with little ones.

There are plenty of other ways to engage the power of touch. Indulge in a professional massage now and then. Rub someone's back. Put a comforting arm around someone's shoulder. Stroke your cat or tickle your dog's tummy. Or walk hand in hand with the man you love. Back home, let that prelude to intimacy lead to lovemaking. That's the best way of all to tap into the healing and rejuvenating miracles of your largest sensory organ—your skin!

There you have it. You've learned all of my Three Rs for Ageless Skin from Within. Promise me—and yourself!—that you'll journal your Releases, Rewards, and Relaxation every day and also continue your daily recording of your Ageless Skin-care Regimen as you move into the last phase of step 2 of my Ageless Skin-Care program.

Now, read on to find out how making the most of every aspect of your looks can not only enhance the appearance of your skin right away but also inspire you to do even more for your skin during the final steps of the program.

6

Spruce Up Your Looks— Make Your Spirit Soar

As you continue step 2 on my program, it's time to start improving your appearance in general. I have seen over and over again that patients who are unhappy with their skin get an instant uplift, which always shows in their skin, when I give them advice about fashion, hair, nails, makeup, and more.

That's one reason that Lucille, the patient I quoted in the introduction of this book, called me a "full-service dermatologist." I have observed that when people are upset about skin issues—particularly the signs of aging—they tend to stop maintaining other aspects of their looks and health. In effect, they give up. They seem to be saying to themselves, "Who am I kidding? I've got wrinkles and age spots. Why bother to try new hairstyles and makeup or buy new clothes?" That's a self-destructive attitude. I set out to identify and change it right away. While I don't think people do themselves a favor by trying to look twentysomething forever, there is no point in aging unattractively. In fact, my take on the adage about "aging gracefully" is that we should fight aging all the way! To that end, I firmly believe there is great therapeutic and skin-rejuvenating value in making the most of your looks overall. Fortunately, a great deal of improvement in your appearance, and therefore the look of your skin, can be achieved almost instantly.

I remember one patient, Emily, who had gained about thirty pounds during menopause. Here's what she told me:

I keep promising myself to lose the weight, but I just can't seem to stick with any diet and exercise program. I just feel so discouraged because I know my hormones and my age are against me. Every time I make up my mind to get serious about weight loss, I end up starving myself all day and then pigging out in front of the refrigerator at night. The next morning, I feel horrible about myself and I give up on the idea of dieting. Well, not totally. I still haven't bought any "fat" clothes. Yuck! I just can't walk into a store and buy "women's" sizes. It's so depressing. So I've been practically living in a couple of outfits that still fit because they have elastic waists. I know they don't look all that great and even my husband very nicely suggested that we have enough in the budget for me to get some new clothes. He didn't say I'm too fat, but of course I knew what he was thinking. That only made me more determined not to buy bigger sizes and to lose the weight, but after one day of my usual starve-and-pig-out routine, I was off my diet again.

⎯◦ ◯ ◦⎯

Pearl: I don't believe in aging gracefully. I believe in fighting it every step of the way.

When Emily had finished pouring out all of this, I nodded in sympathy and told her about my own earlier struggle with weight gain. She looked amazed because I am not at all overweight now. I promised to help her succeed, partly by changing her attitude about herself through my Three Rs. But first, I started by teaching her the Ageless Skin-care Regimen you learned in chapter 2.

Right there in my office, after her first cleansing/moisturizing/sun protection session, I had her look in the mirror. Devoid of the caked-on makeup she had been wearing, she actually looked younger than she had just minutes before. Then I offered her ideas about lighter makeup—with built-in sunscreen of course! I also reviewed bronzers and ways she could use soft colors to accentuate her good features with very little effort. I helped her see that if she stopped making a mask of her face and clogging her skin along the way, her skin would improve and that would put her into a better cycle.

Before she left, I gently suggested that she should take her husband up on his offer of a little money for some flattering clothes. "You're going to lose the weight soon, I promise you," I said. "But in the meantime you'll feel a lot better about yourself and a lot more motivated to succeed with your diet and with your skin-care if you dress so you look your best. Why not get just two or three outfits, maybe those pretty print dresses that have flowing dusters over them or some suits that are tailored to your new curves?" I knew her skin would be less itchy and irritated if she stopped wearing tight clothing, and that she'd look great and not at all matronly. She grinned and said she'd give it some thought.

At her next visit I could really see the difference. She walked taller, she had more colorful clothing that fit better and flattered her figure, and her face was looking great. I could see that she had been ready for a change, which is why she came to me, and she had really taken the advice I gave her to heart. She said, "Doc, you have to write this stuff down. It would make a great book."

She obviously felt much better about herself, and when I went on to teach her the Three Rs, the first Release she recorded in her journal was, "I will stop making myself miserable about gaining weight. I look great even with a few extra pounds." The very happy ending is that she was motivated to go to a nutritionist, and within six months she had pared off all the extra pounds and then some. She gave her "fat clothes" to a thrift shop and invested in some current fashions to show off her trim new silhouette. She was also religious through all of this about following the Ageless Skin-care Regimen and about journaling her Three Rs. Those good skin-care habits, plus some Restalyne treatments—a small miracle you'll learn about in chapter 11—literally transformed her face. She told me that when she went to her fortieth high school reunion, she was voted the class-mate who looked the most like her senior picture.

Emily is not an exception. She is the rule. It does not take much to start a turn in the tide of how you look and take care of yourself. When you begin with your focus on your skin, you will see that the effects go so much deeper and are very rewarding for the skin, body, and mind. This is why the skin is my favorite organ. It is beautiful and sensual and truly a reflection of so much more than what you think you see when you look in the mirror. I remember meeting people in various social situations and thinking they were so beautiful or so

Pearl: Once you've finished your hair and makeup, that should be the last time you look in a mirror until you think you need to freshen up at some point later on. Just carry in your mind the image of yourself as pulled-together and looking great rather than checking yourself out at every opportunity.

ugly, and thinking that their skin looked good or bad. But I noticed that as I got to know them, they started to change in my view. Depending on their mannerisms, their actions, their attitudes, and their confidence, their overall appearance and the look of their skin would change right before my eyes. It's one thing how your skin looks in a concrete sense, but how you project yourself is a different matter entirely. Your demeanor has a dramatic effect on what people think your skin looks like. While my goal is always first and foremost to create and enhance beautiful skin, I also look to enhance the more abstract and esoteric essence of the skin. I know the combination gives the most beautiful and lasting results.

Now let's get to work on making positive changes in how *you* look from top to toe. I can guarantee that your skin will look younger and clearer as a result.

HAIRSTYLES AND COLOR

Hair is part of a dermatologist's specialty. Like your skin, your hair tells your dermatologist a lot about your general health. Dull, lifeless hair is a giveaway that a patient is not in peak physical condition. Shiny, resilient hair speaks of robust good health. Hair contains no nerves or blood, but nutrients are taken from the bloodstream via a papilla at the end of the root. Also, sebaceous glands below the surface of the skin secrete sebum. This fatty substance nourishes the hair. If you improve your lifestyle, which we'll be talking more about in chapters 7 through 10, the changes will be reflected in a healthier head of hair.

However, you can start right now to make the most of your looks with a truly becoming hairstyle and color. As a general rule, medium to short hairstyles have an uplifting effect on the face. Longer styles tend to emphasize wrinkles, and really long hair is usually too girlish for anyone with mature skin. The exception is long hair pulled away from the face and into a French twist or chignon. In fact, catching your hair in a clip or elastic actually gives you a temporary face-lift! On the other hand, if you opt for a close-cropped style, you'll have a full head of gray hair fairly quickly. Plenty of stylish women look wonderful with well-cut short or medium-length gray or white hair, especially when they pick a new palette of makeup and wardrobe colors to enhance their silver-haired image.

Still, you may decide to color your hair even if you keep it fairly short. The standard advice is to go a shade or two lighter than your natural color, but not to go all the way to blond unless that's really your hair color. However, everyone is different. Get the advice of a good colorist, and also trust your instincts about what will make you look and feel great. The good news is that today's hair coloring products condition your hair and give you natural-looking nuances.

Overall, my advice to patients who come to me for skin rejuvenation—and now my advice to you as well—is that a flattering and up-to-date hairstyle will go a long way toward giving both your face and your mood a lift. Try it and see!

HAIR LOSS

One of the most difficult problems a patient comes in with is hair loss. Many women experience occasional temporary thinning of the hair, known as telogen effluvium, usually caused by physiologic stressors

Pearl: On a bad hair day, try a loose ponytail and finish with outsized hoop or dangle earrings. Gorgeous!

such as childbirth, major surgery, or serious injuries. In those cases, the growth patterns of all the hairs have become synchronized with one another so that all the hairs grow and fall out at the same time. Actually, any kind of stress can affect hair growth due to "fight or flight," an auto-response system to stress or trauma. When faced with increased levels of stress or trauma, the body automatically redirects the flow of the blood, and with it oxygen and nutrients, to areas it considers vital for responding to the stress. It simultaneously with-draws from areas it considers nonessential, such as the skin and hair. This response constricts the capillaries, causing a lack of oxygen and nutrient uptake, as well as poor vitamin and nutrient assimilation for the skin, nails, and hair follicles. However, the hair eventually grows back, and the cycles of each hair return to their normal and healthy unsynchronized growth patterns.

Even so, every day I see women who bring in Baggies filled with hair or who complain that they have been losing hair for years. Meanwhile, when I look at their scalps, I still see a full head of hair. They often tell me that they agree they still have plenty of hair, but they are concerned they will go bald in the future. I do my best to re-assure them that while I cannot foresee what will be, nothing I see now tells me they will go bald, ever. Some women do have thinning hair, and they look for every possible reason. They get all their hor-mones checked, they have thyroid tests even though they have no symptoms of thyroid disease, they worry about everything under the sun. They are terrified that they will go bald. Some have a family his-tory of hair loss, but most don't.

Genetics also determine the shape and texture of your hair be-cause you inherit the shape of the follicles. Straight hair grows from straight hair follicles and thus has a smooth, shiny appearance. This is because its cuticle (outer layer) emerges tight and smooth from the round-shaped hair follicle. In the same way, wavy hair grows from a kinky-shaped follicle and grows at a slight angle to the scalp. Like-wise, coarse hair emerges from elongated oval follicles that have a bend to them.

When the hair curves, as is the case with medium to coarse and frizzy hair, the hair's cuticle lifts, causing its shinglelike microscopic layers to lift. In these instances, the cuticle is permanently lifted and is more likely than straight hair to be brittle, frizzy, and lacking in shine. Curly hair also has poor porosity and lacks the natural ability to absorb and retain moisture. Also note that poor scalp hygiene, residues from chemical services, buildup from conventional ingredients, and follicular debris can alter follicle shape and the direction in which the hair strand grows out of the follicle.

To reassure you, I want you to remember that normal shedding of hair is about 100 to 150 a day. Hair has three cycles of growth. Normally, each hair on your head grows about a half inch per month for between two and six years and then falls out. Then a new hair starts growing out of the same follicle.

Stages of Hair Growth

Anagen

This is the growing phase. It can last from months to years, depending on the part of the body and genetic influences. The longer the anagen cycle, the longer the hair will grow before it falls out. About 90 percent of all hair is in this cycle at any given time.

Catagen

This is the resting phase. It lasts about three to four months. Approximately 8 to 10 percent of hair is in this cycle at any given time.

Telogen

This is the shedding phase. It lasts a few weeks before the hair starts to grow again. About 1 to 2 percent of hair is in this cycle at any given time.

If all of your hair were in the same cycle at the same time, all the hair would move from the growing to the resting to the falling-out phase

Major Causes of Thinning Hair

- **Genetic predisposition**
- **Stress and trauma**
- **Nutrition and diet**
- **Autoimmune conditions**
- **Hormonal conditions**
- **Medications**
- **Environmental toxins**

A few of the vitamins and minerals crucial for healthy hair growth include:

- **Niacin (Vitamin B$_3$):** A component of the vitamin B complex, niacin is essential for cellular metabolic processes. Niacin can also function as a vasodilator, enhancing blood circulation of the scalp and stimulating the metabolism of hair follicles. Found in: cheese, chicken, fish, beans, wheat bran and whole-grain wheat products, nuts.
- **Folic acid (Vitamin B$_9$):** A water-soluble vitamin, folic acid helps the body with cellular replication, growth, and protein synthesis, and aids in the formation of genetic material within body cells. Folic acid has also been shown to support healthy skin and hair production. Found in: beans, green leafy vegetables, wheat germ, fruits.

- **Biotin:** Also a member of the B-complex group of vitamins, biotin appears to help metabolize fatty and amino acids, which are valuable growth factors in numerous bodily processes, including the production of hair, skin, and nails. Found in: egg yolks, organ meats, soybeans, fish, whole grains.
- **Calcium:** Ususally associated with the formation of healthy bones and teeth, calcium is also a major component of healthy, strong hair. Found in: dairy products; green, leafy vegetables; tofu; almonds; enriched flour products.
- **Zinc:** Zinc helps stabilize cell membranes to strengthen their defenses against free radical attacks. It also assists in immune functions and cellular growth/development. Found in: seafood, red meats, beans, yogurt, dairy products, wheat germ.
- **Coenzymes:** One of science's greatest discoveries against the body's aging processes, coenzymes—especially coenzyme Q_{10} nutrients—have been known to dramatically help reverse signs of aging in hair, skin, and nails by encouraging cellular turnover. They also promote a healthy scalp/skin environment, which may extend the life cycle of hair.

I like a line of products from NIOXIN Research Laboratories, Inc. It was founded in 1987 by Eva Graham and is devoted to skin care for the scalp.

together and you would go bald every few years. Fortunately, these hair growth cycles are not synchronized, but hair does fall out at a rate of 1 to 2 percent per day. Depending on how much hair you have and how long it is, this can look like a lot of hair. But that same amount, more or less, is growing back at the same time, so there is no cause for worry. And even if you experience hair loss as a result of stress, the hair will eventually grow back.

Sophie writes:

I was always a very highly motivated person so when I had the opportunity to keep moving up the partnership ladder at my law firm, I kept putting off having children until one day my doctor said now or never. I was over forty by then, but we were lucky to conceive a child after only two months of trying. My pregnancy was uneventful and after the delivery I nursed during my three-month maternity leave and even after I went back to work I pumped breast milk. I felt thrilled about the baby, but I'll have to admit that I was very stressed. Right about that time, I was absolutely mortified when my hair started to come out in what felt like clumps. There was hair everywhere. It clogged the shower drain, it was all over my pillow, and the hair on my head was looking thinner and thinner. I could even see down to my scalp in a few areas. I ran to my dermatologist. Dr. Day reassured me that this was a "normal" process that occurs in many women a few months after childbirth and that all or most of the hair would come back. She even showed me areas where hair had started to grow in already. I felt a little better. I still hated it but I could see that it would pass. In the meantime, Dr. Day suggested that I should consider investing in a good wig, and also try wearing stylish scarves and turbans and hats when I wasn't in a mood for the wig. That boosted my morale like you wouldn't believe!

Other types of hair loss are due to hormonal, genetic, or immune influence. Alopecia areata is a condition where you see round patches of hair loss but with no scarring. It can occur on any part of the body. For some unknown reason, the body mounts an immune attack against certain hair follicles. Sometimes, fortunately rarely, it attacks all the hair follicles. In these cases, all the hair on the body from head to toe is lost. It can occur at any age, ethnicity, or gender. When it occurs in a patchy fashion, injections of cortisone into the areas often help the hair grow back. While we don't know the cause, the general consensus is that stress is an exacerbating factor.

Another type of hair loss is related to polycystic ovary disease. This condition is slowly being better defined and more efficiently treated. There are several signs and symptoms, such as irregular periods, excessive weight gain, and severe acne, among others. Women with PCO are at higher risk for diabetes and other medical concerns and should be treated and followed regularly. Treatment usually involves oral contraceptives and other drugs to balance the hormones. Sometimes medicines used for people with type 2 diabetes are also used as treatment for PCO.

A much more common type of hair loss is called androgenic alopecia. This is a genetic form of hair loss and is just about as common in women as it is in men, although the pattern is different for women than what we typically see in male-pattern hair loss. Women don't tend to go completely bald as men do. We keep the frontal hairline and thin out right behind it. There are two types of general patterns that we see. One is called patterned alopecia, where the loss is mostly at the front and top of the scalp, and the other is called nonpatterned alopecia, where the loss is more diffuse. There are some ways of slowing the process, but it is what it is. Some day we will figure a way to clone hair so that everyone can have as much hair as they want. In the meantime, the Food and Drug Administration (FDA) has approved a topical medication called monoxidil 2%, sold as Rogaine, to treat female alopecia. An estimated one-quarter of female alopecia sufferers experience new hair growth as a result of the Rogaine treatments, which cost about $600 a year for twice-daily applications to the scalp. The other 75 percent of affected women may find that the treatments slow down or even stop the loss of hair. But if treatments are ended, hair loss resumes. I think that the men's strength, which is 5 percent, works better, but it does have a higher risk of causing hair to grow on other parts of the body, including the face. Another hair loss medication, Propecia, does not work for women and is in fact dangerous for women even to touch if they are pregnant since it affects hormones that are important for the developing penis of a male fetus. In other words, don't take or touch this drug if you are pregnant or in your childbearing years.

One drug that has been tried with some success for women—but again not women planning pregnancy—is spironolactone. It affects a specific hormone receptor and can be useful even in women who have no overt signs of hormonal imbalance.

An excellent treatment for certain types of androgenic alopecia is hair transplants. This is a procedure in which rows of hair, along with the underlying skin, are taken from unaffected areas at the back of the scalp, called the donor site, and inserted into the balding areas. The rows are divided into single hairs or into units of two to four hairs. When the skin at the donor site is then sewn or stapled back together, there is merely a fine line that remains that is covered by the surrounding hair. There is a very low risk of scarring and skin infection when the procedure is done correctly, so be sure to choose a board-certified doctor who comes highly recommended. Several sessions are usually needed, and the total cost is in the neighborhood of $3,000 and up. Results are natural-looking and permanent. A final warning: The use of hair implants made of artificial fibers has not been approved by the FDA because of the unacceptably high rate of infection.

If you would rather not have a hair transplant, consider wearing a wig or hairpiece. It is important to make sure that these place as little tension as possible on the scalp so that you don't end up pulling out the hair you have left. However, my feeling is that since hair loss in women is unacceptable in society, you should do whatever you can to minimize the appearance of hair loss, even if there is some potential for damage to the remaining hair.

Another option is hair weaving and hair extensions, also called hair fusion. These are techniques which attach locks of human hair to your own hair. Be sure to find a hair salon/hair-care expert who specializes in this treatment since, if done improperly, it can cause scarring and worsening of the hair loss.

Finally, I like a product called Toppik. It is a powder, not a colorant, which binds to the hair and minimizes the appearance of baldness/thinning in the affected areas.

FACIAL HAIR

Excessive hair growth on a woman's face can indicate an underlying medical condition involving the pituitary gland, adrenal gland, or ovaries. If you have coarse hair on your upper lip or chin, bring this up with your doctor. Most women, though, have some facial hair, more like peach fuzz, such as a light mustache after puberty and at least a few chin whiskers later in life. That's not cause for concern. However, it's not what our society considers attractive! You've probably already experimented with some form of facial hair removal, particularly if you have light skin and dark hair. Do-it-yourself methods may work for you, including tweezing, shaving, and over-the-counter depilatories. Yet the drawbacks of these solutions are that they have to be repeated regularly, even daily, and they may irritate the skin and thus cause unsightly redness. Waxing is another possibility you may have tried, either at home or in a salon, but again the results are not permanent and irritation is possible.

One method that gives more lasting results is electrolysis. It is considered permanent, but maintenance treatments are usually required over time. The procedure has been around for more than one hundred years and works by damaging hair follicles with tiny jolts of electricity. Electrolysis should be done by a certified practitioner. The cost is about $40 to $60 and up per half-hour session. The drawback is that there is some risk of discoloration and scarring, and multiple treatments are necessary. Electrolysis is also painful and not all the hair can be addressed at every session. This is probably the best option for people with just a few hairs or who have white or blond hair.

All the methods I've mentioned so far for facial hair removal have downsides. The good news is that there is an excellent method called laser hair removal that is quick and long lasting, although not necessarily permanent even though the FDA has approved the laser treatments as permanent. However, the hair that regrows is finer and softer and it grows much more slowly than before the treatments. There is only mild discomfort during the treatments.

Laser hair removal is only performed by dermatologists. The average cost is $150 for the upper lip. Imagine waking up every morning with a smooth, hair-free complexion! For that matter, imagine feeling free to kiss the person you love any time of day or night without worrying about stubble.

Whether you opt for laser hair removal, or you choose another method, do get rid of that facial hair. I can guarantee you'll feel better about yourself and more excited than ever about following my Ageless Skin-Care program.

NAILS

Your nails, like your skin, can tell your dermatologist a great deal about your health, including the possibility of serious problems, such as kidney and liver disease. Far more common, though, are symptoms like weak, splitting nails that indicate a patient is probably not getting enough good nutrition, water, exercise, and sound sleep. Beyond that, in my practice I always note whether or not a patient has well-groomed nails. It doesn't matter if she does her own manicure or gets a professional one, or if she prefers light shades of polish or bright shades or French nails. Her cared-for nails let me know that she's in a frame of mind that allows her to be good to herself and care about her looks. But if her cuticles are ragged, her nails have been nibbled on, or her polish is chipped, I know that she's worried or sad or simply suffering from low self-esteem, or maybe just has too much going on in her life and needs to prioritize.

When I see a pattern of unkempt nails, I do a bit of questioning. I often find that the problem stems directly from a patient's dissatisfaction with her skin, which is what brought her to me in the first place. That's when I encourage her to make immediate improvement in the look of her nails as a step toward feeling better about herself, even as I help her improve her skin. When a patient takes my advice and comes back for her next visit with prettier nails, the smile on her face tells me that her self-esteem has already gotten a big boost. And as you know by now, the success of my Ageless Skin-Care program relies on taking full advantage of the inextricable connection between all aspects of our being—mind, body, and spirit. That's why I encourage you, like my patients, to give yourself an instant lift by starting right now to take good care of your nails.

Dermatologists specialize in nails, just as we do in skin and hair. I find the medical aspects of nails fascinating. Nails consist of the nail plate, which is the part you see; the cuticle, which is the tissue that covers the base of the plate; the nail bed, which is the skin beneath the nail plate; the nail folds, the skin that supports the nails on all three sides; the lunula, which is the "moon" at the base of the plate; and the matrix, which is under the cuticle. It is usually most visible on the thumb and index fingernails. The lunula and the matrix in the area of the cuticle are where the new and dividing nail cells are that

Pearl: Your cuticles are your friends.
Don't cut them off.

make up the nails you see. As they grow, they get pushed up, and they stop dividing. If you damage the matrix or the lunula, this can lead to scarring, which can cause a permanent deformity of the nail. This is why it is better to avoid picking at your cuticles.

You should also be careful not to let any manicurist cut your cuticles because if they get infected, there can be scarring which can lead to permanent damage to the nail. Also, some people inadvertently damage their own nails because they have what is called a "habit tic." They unconsciously press on their cuticles, usually on the cuticle of the thumbnail with the index finger. This resulting "habit tic deformity" looks like an indentation along the middle of the nail from the cuticle often to the tip of the nail. I can usually observe a patient with this condition pressing on her cuticle without realizing it right in my office. The nail often recovers if she can teach herself to stop touching the cuticle.

Nails are made of a type of keratin, the protein that also makes up skin and hair. Fingernails grow faster than toenails, and the rate of growth is affected by such factors as age, gender, and the season of the year. Nails usually grow faster when you're young, if you're male, and if it's the summer. The nails on your dominant hand grow faster than those on the other hand. Nails also grow faster and stronger if you're in good general health. So treat yourself to a manicure at a reliable nail salon, but don't forget to treat your whole self well while you're at it.

EXCESSIVE SWEATING

The medical term for this condition is hyperhidrosis. If you have it, you know it! Either your palms or your armpits or your feet, or all three, drip with embarrassing amounts of sweat, especially when you're nervous or excited. I've had patients with hyperhidrosis who tell me they are afraid to shake hands with people and that this has adversely affected their career advancement, since they often won't even go for job interviews or take positions where they have to do any public speaking for fear of sweating through their jackets during their speech. It also has profound effects on their social life. They are too embarrassed to hold hands or wear certain outfits due to the unsightly sweating. Many patients tell me that in a high-pressure situation, such as a top-level corporate meeting, their clothes are soaked with perspiration from their armpits. As for feet, the problems stemming from hyperhidrosis include uncomfortably soggy socks and shoes and the resulting unpleasant odor.

Over-the-counter antiperspirants usually prove ineffective for hyperhidrosis sufferers. However, several prescription treatments are available. One is a prescription topical antiperspirant, such as Drysol, which contains a higher concentration of the same active ingredient found in over-the-counter antiperspirants. This is effective for a lot of people, at least for a while, although it can be very irritating to the skin. There is also an oral prescription medication called glycopyrrolate, or under the brand name of Robinul, but it has uncomfortable side effects, such as dry mouth and dry eyes. It is sometimes used in combination with a beta-blocker called propranolol, more commonly used for control of high blood pressure. Blood pressure should be monitored regularly while on this drug. Another option is a procedure called iontophoresis, which uses electrical currents. This cannot be done on the underarms due to the curve of the area, and it has to be repeated regularly, often two to three times per week to maintain results. Treatments take half an hour or longer, which makes them very time-consuming. Finally, there is a surgical procedure called a sympathectomy, which is the surgical clipping or severing of the nerves that supply the sweat glands of the desired area, usually performed by a neurosurgeon.

Another treatment that has been used with some success is biofeedback. Since this type of sweating starts with the brain, the idea is that you can modify and control, at least to some extent, the effect your subconscious mind has on your sweat glands.

None of these options are ideal, and the surgical option is not

Pearl: My recommendation to my patients who sweat excessively is the most up-to-date, safe, and effective treatment: Botox injections.

without risks and side effects. My recommendation to my patients is the most up-to-date, safe, and effective treatment: Botox injections. There's detailed information about Botox in chapter 11, but in brief, the drug temporarily weakens the muscles involved in producing sweat. The effect lasts for several months. I've helped nervous brides, job applicants on their way to interviews, performers, speakers with stage fright, and plenty of other people who needed to know that hyperhidrosis wouldn't suddenly mortify them. Believe me, their newfound peace of mind showed on their faces virtually overnight! If you are a hyperhidrosis sufferer, I hope you'll make an appointment with a dermatologist right away to get Botox injections.

Peter writes:

I am a Broadway actor. I am in the public eye, and I need to wear certain costumes on stage. My problem is that nothing worked. I tried the stuff in the stores. Nothing. I tried Drysol. I got the most itchy rash and redness, and it took a week of topical cortisone cream to make it better. When Dr. Day told me about Botox, I thought she was confused as to why I was there. She assured me she understood and that Botox treatments would help me. I said sign me up. She did about twenty small pinpricks under each arm. I barely knew she was doing anything. The next day the improvement started. I was amazed. The day after, it was even better. I can wear things I never could before. It has affected parts of my life in ways I could never even have imagined. She warned me I might have some weakness of my hand, like trouble opening a jar, but I had nothing. I go in once a year when the sweating starts to come back. It is my favorite place to go. I know I am going to get results that I will love.

WARDROBE

Remember how I suggested that Emily, my overweight patient, would feel better if she stopped squeezing into her "thin" clothes and bought some more attractive flowing dresses, or outfits tailored to her body instead? I discuss fashion and color with my patients all the time, when it is appropriate. Some people are naturally more comfortable in color while others prefer earth tones. A combination is ideal. In addition to advice about color, I might look at you and explain that a higher neckline would be a flattering way to conceal the sun-damaged skin on your neck. Or I might point out that brighter colors such as magenta and turquoise and purple would not only lift your mood but also make your skin look younger and more vibrant.

I'm sure you've heard the now-classic poem that begins "When I'm an old woman, I shall wear purple." There is so much truth in that poem! Aging doesn't have to mean "hiding" in bland, neutral, boring clothes. Rejuvenate your wardrobe, and you'll look and feel younger right away! And the very act of making yourself look better and younger by dressing with some panache will put a twinkle in your eye and soften the look of wrinkles. Different skin colors look better with different colored fabrics. I try to help guide my patients when they indicate they are receptive to the advice.

SHOES

High heels make your legs look marvelous, and I'm all for wearing them on occasion. But pinched and painful feet will give you a pinched and pained expression that will in turn engrave lines on your face. Make a practice of wearing sturdy, comfortable walking shoes and bringing your stilettos along to put on when you're ready to meet your public. I love my heels and I wear them in the office at least a few days a week. But I always have my walking shoes for my two-mile walk home from the office. My feet would not forgive me if I tried that in my heels. I did try it once, so I can tell you from experience that it is not a good idea!

MAKEUP

A lot of women cake on too much makeup in an effort to mask wrinkles and imperfections, or choose the wrong color. For instance, darker-skinned women may opt for shades too light for them in an effort to lighten up a bit, or women may choose shades that are too warm or cool for their natural skin tones. That's a mistake. Look for a luminous, moist foundation with sunscreen protection that will give you a smoother, glowing look. Also, try out different eye shadows to see which ones stay put, rather than slithering into creases and folds. And take advantage of the new lines of long-lasting lipsticks that don't smear or run into fine lines around the mouth. In addition, pay attention to your coloring. If you've decided to let your hair go silver, change your makeup palette accordingly. Why not get a consultation from a makeup artist, either at a department store, salon, or spa? There's nothing like professional advice to steer you toward just the right makeup textures and shades to make the most of your looks.

You might also consider micropigmentation, sometimes called permanent makeup. This procedure is performed by board-certified

> *Pearl:* Makeup is not bad for your skin as long as you cleanse and moisturize morning and night. You can wear makeup seven days a week if you want to.

permanent makeup artists and can offer beautiful, lasting results that are liberating. You wake up and are ready to go. You can always add makeup as a supplement for special occasions. People who have no eyebrows due to too much plucking over the years often find that it is difficult to draw the brows on just right every day. Also, going swimming or getting caught in a downpour can wash off the penciled-in brows and that can be embarrassing. Similarly, some people lose eyebrows and or eyelashes due to various conditions, or to treatments such as chemotherapy, and would benefit from these treatments as well. For others micropigmentation is a matter of convenience and "liberation." If you wear your eyeliner the same way every day, it is wonderful to get it done permanently. This way you will wake up every day looking the way you like.

EYEWEAR

In spite of Dorothy Parker's warning that "men seldom make passes at girls who wear glasses," you can look wonderful in glasses. Just be sure you pick an up-to-date style that's flattering as well as functional. If all you need is reading glasses, consider having some fun with a batch of them in fashion colors. For those who need more than just-for-reading vision correction, some may prefer contact lenses.

Today's offerings are comfortable, disposable, and not terribly expensive. You can even get colored lenses if you'd like to "try on" a new eye color, perhaps to go with your newly colored hair or your silver-haired look. Talk about an instant makeover!

Another contact lens option, if you're both nearsighted and farsighted, is "monovision." Let's say your left eye is better than your right when it comes to distance vision, but your right eye is better at close-up tasks such as reading. You will get a lens that corrects for distance vision to use in your left eye and a lens that corrects for close work to use in your right eye. Your eyes adjust almost instantly so that you can read and use the computer without glasses, and drive and watch movies without glasses as well. If you're just getting to the point where you need reading glasses, this trick will keep you from giving that fact away. You'll be able to read small print on restaurant menus, for instance, without whipping out those telltale "readers."

If you do wear contact lenses, learn to put them in and take them out without pulling on the delicate skin around your eyes, as I already mentioned in chapter 2. Also, be extra careful to moisturize your eye area and use sun protection. Laugh lines around your eyes will be more visible if you're wearing contacts than if you were wearing glasses.

You might also consider laser eye surgery to correct myopia (nearsightedness), hyperopia (genetic farsightedness), presbyopia (age-related farsightedness), or astigmatism (distorted vision). Of all the surgical corrective techniques available, laser surgery is the one recommended by the American Academy of Ophthalmology. An estimated 20 percent of the country's ophthalmologists are trained in laser surgery. Be sure you research a potential doctor's qualifications and success rate before choosing this procedure.

According to the Food and Drug Administration, 5 percent of patients still need glasses for nearsightedness after surgery, and another 15 percent need them for driving. However, another 5 percent actually have worse vision after the surgery. Obviously, having laser surgery is a big decision that is not without risks. Just remember that

Pearl: If a man tells you that he loves the "natural look" and you shouldn't wear makeup, ignore him. Women (and men!) in all cultures have been enhancing their looks with cosmetics since the beginning of time. Think of makeup as an art form, not as artifice.

if your vision needs correcting, find a solution that plays up your looks, gives you confidence, and makes you smile when you catch a glimpse of yourself in the mirror. Your reward will be a radiance that will have people remarking about what lovely skin you have!

HEALTHY TEETH

I can plump the lips. I can soften the lines around the mouth. I can smooth the skin of the face. After all of this, I look and see a mouthful of crooked or yellow teeth or front teeth that stick out or in and make the mouth seem smaller. The teeth have a very large impact on the attractiveness and youthfulness of the face. The health of teeth plays a large role in the beauty of the face. A beautiful, healthy smile changes the look of the whole face for the better. As the wife of a dentist, I've looked at many photos that prove this. See what I mean in figures 6.1 and 6.2 on page 149. For more photos, go to www.dentistnyc.com.

It is very important to brush your teeth at least twice every day, and brushing after every meal and snack is better. Flossing every day is even more important. A number of recent studies have shown that flossing on a regular basis can add two or more years to your life expectancy. This is because a buildup of the bacteria that cause periodontal disease can trigger an immune reaction called hyperinflammation which in turn can lead to heart disease and stroke. If you floss daily, you'll get to keep your teeth and in all probability you'll live longer to enjoy them! Not bad! Not only that, but if you don't end up needing to have teeth pulled, you'll avoid the sunken cheek look that is so aging. If you find flossing difficult or unpleasant, try using disposable floss picks. I carry several in my purse and slip into the ladies' room to use one after a restaurant meal.

In addition, if you never had braces as a child, it's not too late to have your teeth straightened. The good news is that you don't have to do it with braces. Although adult orthodontia is becoming increasingly popular these days, with an estimated 20 percent of orthodontic patients now over the age of eighteen, the problem is that this shifting of the teeth can lead to loss of bone and the need for a lifelong retainer to prevent the teeth from moving back. That's why, if you do choose to give yourself a brand-new smile, I recommend that you consider porcelain veneers instead of braces. Ask your orthodontist about them. Veneers are a very simple and quick way to get the teeth you want without the pain and without the wait. The results are much more predictable than with traditional braces, and you can have teeth that are a shade or two whiter than the teeth you have. Be sure to see a prosthodontist or a cosmetic dentist since these treatments are very technique-dependent and performing the procedure is an art. Once you have your new smile, your face will light up with confidence and that will enhance everything you're doing to rejuvenate your skin.

Congratulations! You've reached the end of step 2 of my Ageless Skin-Care program. I'll wager that you've already been getting compliments, although many people may not be able to put a finger on

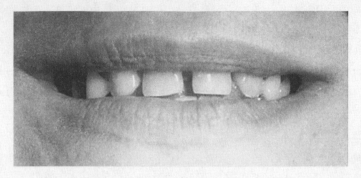

FIGURE 6.1
Misaligned teeth, providing little lip support,
making the lips appear thinner.

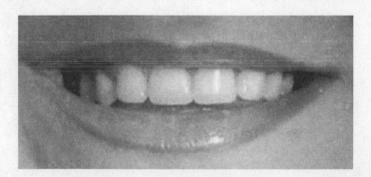

FIGURE 6.2
The same teeth two days later after the application
of veneers. Perfectly aligned teeth provide
greater lip support, increasing the
appearance of lip volume.

exactly why you're suddenly looking so vibrant. You've probably been hearing some version of "You look younger than the last time I saw you!" You can verify this for yourself by recalculating your score on the Skin Aging Test. I'm certain you'll find that your scores on Skin Age Factors have already improved significantly.

It's time to move on to step 3, during which you'll continue to improve your scores on your Skin Age Factors. Turn the page to begin my easy and energizing Ageless Skin Diet and Exercise Program.

The Ageless Skin Diet and Exercise Program

7

How Eating Right Benefits Your Skin

What you eat affects every organ in your body, and your skin is no exception. You may think that as long as you are using an expensive skin cream with a bunch of ingredients with scientific-sounding names, your skin will be properly nourished. Nope, not true. While a skin cream may provide a number of important substances, it can never replace proper skin nutrition from within. But I want to assure you that as I sit here writing while sipping on a delicious smoothie, I can tell you with confidence and scientific backing that eating right is not a punishment. Good nutrition that helps you toward your goal of youthful skin does not mean eating bland food that tastes like cardboard. Food that's good for your skin can be delicious as well as satisfying for both your body and soul. I promise you that when you follow my Skin-Friendly Food Regimen you'll find in chapter 8, your kitchen will be redolent with spices and herbs such as rosemary, oregano, nutmeg, and cinnamon. And your table will be laden with wholesome, colorful dishes that will tempt not only you but also your entire family. Better yet, the food will taste terrific, without your having to spend all day sweating over a hot stove—although your family may think you did!

AVOID "EMPTY CALORIES"

More and more research is being done that shows the beneficial effects of certain food in slowing or even reversing the aging process of many organ systems, including the skin. It is still often very confusing, since the science is in many ways so young when it comes to fats, sugars, vitamins, and hormones and their effects on the body. What was considered so good or bad for you just a few years ago may now be considered the opposite. This has served to reduce many people's confidence in the science of nutrition. However, one basic fact remains as it has been—food should have a value besides simply calories. It should provide nutrients that your body requires. This is why you should try to convince yourself as a rational, motivated adult to give up or at least minimize consumption of foods that contain only unhealthy fats and sugar without any vitamins, minerals, and protein. You know what these are—the desserts and fried foods that may taste good but are so bad for your body and your skin.

DR. DAY'S TEN COMMANDMENTS FOR THE CARE AND FEEDING OF YOUR SKIN

Now I want to share with you my Ten Commandments. They will help you get the most out of the skin-friendly recipes and meal plans you'll find in chapter 8.

1. Eat Raw Fruits and Vegetables

Fruits and vegetables are a superior source of skin-enhancing nutrients including antioxidants, and you'll really reap their benefits if you avoid cooking away much of what nature put into that apple or carrot or bowl of blueberries. Remember, too, that the skins of many fruits and vegetables, including apples, pears, and tomatoes, are chockful of nutrients and give you much-needed fiber. There's nothing wrong with indulging in healthy smoothies now and then, but whenever possible, bite into a whole fruit. By the same token, it is wonderful to steam your veggies to go with a hot meal or cook tomatoes to make a sauce, but make sure you also munch on fresh, raw cauliflower, broccoli, carrots, spinach, and grape tomatoes for lunch and for snacks. Your skin, and figure, will thank you for it!

2. Don't Overcook Any Food

Overcooking, boiling, and deep-frying deplete food of essential nutrients and antioxidants and raise the amount of skin-damaging oxidative by-products. Once you master nutrient-preserving cooking techniques such as steaming and broiling, you'll find that your food tastes far better than it did when it was subjected to too much heat, or too much time in the oven or frying pan.

3. Keep Your Skin Hydrated

When skin is well hydrated, it is more plump and resilient. This is due, at least in part, to an ingredient in the skin called hyaluronic acid. The job of hyaluronic acid in the skin is to hold water. When there is adequate water from inside and out, the skin looks healthier and more vibrant and is less prone to wrinkles. It is important to drink lots of fluids throughout the day for best results. You've probably heard that drinking six to eight glasses of water a day is a good idea, but you may need more or less, depending on your activity level. Coffee and sodas do not count as sources of water because they contain caffeine, which is a diuretic, meaning that they draw water out of your system and your skin. Also, try to control your salt intake since even if you have normal blood pressure, an excess of salt in the diet will lead to water retention and will make your skin, especially around the eyes, puffier. If you've had too much salt, drink lots of water to flush the salt out of your body. Two of my favorite drinks are naturally sparkling water (not seltzer) with a twist of lemon or lime, and green tea as part of my daily fluid intake. What I do is make a large pitcher of water. I add lemon, lime, orange, or cucumber slices and let them "marinate" overnight. The water has a refreshing flavor that is not overpowering and not sweet. I can easily go through a pitcher a day. I often refill a few times. The flavor really lasts, even if you don't change the fruit or cucumber for a week. In addition, start each day with a glass of water with 1 teaspoon of fresh-squeezed lemon.

I also use the water as a base in many of the recipes in chapter 3.

4. Avoid Simple Sugars

Simple sugars, like table sugar and refined carbohydrates, are bad for your skin, just as they are bad for the rest of your body, because they are empty calories. If you fill up on them, you are depriving your skin of food with skin-boosting nutrients. Also, if you eat too much of simple sugars and other simple carbohydrates, or foods with a high glycemic index, you increase your risk of weight gain, lower your energy levels, and can incur type 2 diabetes and other health problems. All of this will show up as unhealthy, prematurely aging skin. Meals that produce a less dramatic rise of blood sugar are far better for the digestion of carbohydrates, and therefore better for the health of your skin. Generally, if choosing among nutritionally equivalent alternatives, the food with lower glycemic effect is what you should pick.

5. Jump-Start Your Metabolism

If you eat the same number of calories and exercise the same amount every day, your body will adjust and your metabolism will be set to a certain level. This is why people stop losing weight when they are on low-calorie diets for periods of more than a few weeks. Their metabolism slows down. They are left hungry and frustrated because for all their efforts, the weight still won't fall off beyond a point. This leads to yo-yo dieting where you repeatedly gain and lose the same ten or fifteen pounds. When that happens, the skin is repeatedly stretched so that it sags when weight is lost. As you age, your skin loses resilience—the ability to "bounce back"—so on-again-off-again dieting can lead to jowls, bags under the eyes, and droopy eyelids.

On the other hand, if you eat more food than usual on a given day or at a given meal, your metabolism will actually increase to burn the extra energy it was given. Then on the next day or at the next meal if you go back to your usual regimen, or even eat a little less, or exercise a little more, you will see that you will either lose weight or at least not gain any. This is a great trick for getting your metabolism jump-started. You are challenging your metabolism in a controlled way by varying the amount of calories over time.

6. Eat Plenty of Fiber-Rich Foods

Fiber used to be considered a basically useless filler because it's not a nutrient. But now we know that fiber reduces the risk of many serious health conditions, including heart disease, diabetes, obesity, colon cancer, and hemorrhoids. Fiber also makes for good digestion and elimination, which helps keep your skin looking vibrant and healthy.

By some estimates, the average American eats only about one-third of the amount of fiber needed daily for peak health. Be sure you include whole grains, especially bran, in your diet every day and that you eat fruits whole so that you'll get enough fiber.

7. Strike a Healthy Balance

Don't fall for diet fads that ask you to eat an inordinate amount of one type of food while limiting others. Every day, your skin needs a sensible balance of nutritious fare from all the food groups: grains and cereals; vegetables and fruits; dairy products; and meat, fish, nuts, and beans. Choose from a variety of colorful foods. That's age-old wisdom that you probably remember from grade school, but it is still the basis of healthy eating that will give your skin the youthful glow you want. And remember, topical skin care products can do only so much for you. They can't counteract the effects of nutritional deficiencies!

8. Stop Looking for a Miracle Diet

There is no magic diet out there that rescues you from the need to consume the right amount of calories for your weight and age. Whether you try low-carb or low-fat or vegetarian or any other fad or theory that comes along, the laws of physics still apply. A calorie is a measurement of heat. Your body burns food as fuel. If you consume too much fuel, it will be stored in your body as fat. True, the popular low-carb/high-fat diets can speed up weight loss because they manipulate the body's metabolic pathways. However, this can backfire on you, especially if you don't follow the diets exactly.

In my experience, I have found that any diet that calls for extremes either in terms of what you do eat or what you don't eat is not only not realistic but also not safe over time. The result is unhealthy skin. Also, remember that even extreme, basically unbalanced diets acknowledge that you can't "eat all you want" or stuff yourself and still lose weight. My desire is for you to be able to become more in tune with your body so you can make choices that are right for you. There are times, and days, your body will need to eat more and days when you are simply not very hungry. Your metabolism will adjust to those ups and downs. You don't need to think about it. You just need to be able listen to your body, to teach yourself to make choices that are right for you, and to stop when you are full.

9. Indulge But Don't Overindulge

Do you love chocolate? Is ice cream your favorite treat? Are you a cookie monster? Then don't deprive yourself entirely of your personal comfort food. You'll only end up caving in and gobbling more than you should at some point. Actually, chocolate, especially dark chocolate, is good for you in reasonable amounts. And the idea that chocolate is bad for your skin, especially if you have acne, is a myth. Research has shown that dark chocolate can help lower blood pressure, boost your brain power, and may also act as an aphrodisiac—which must be why it's traditionally been a lover's gift! And as for other sweets and even fatty or salty snacks such as potato chips and pretzels, if you discipline yourself to enjoy a moderate amount now and then, there will be no harm done. Remember, one cookie or one candy bar won't make you fat or give you acne or spoil the youthful glow of your skin. It's poor food choices on a regular basis that will do you in!

Pearl: One cookie won't make you fat or spoil your skin, so let yourself enjoy!

10. Experiment in the Kitchen

I love to cook, and I love to experiment with recipes that I've collected over time. I encourage you to do the same. I am constantly modifying recipes by substituting sweeteners for sugar, reducing the amount of skin-damaging salt, using healthy alternatives to butter, and amping up the flavor and aroma by adding spices and herbs. For a while, I was a dash-of-this-and-dash-of-that cook, which meant that I was the only one who really knew what I had done to a recipe to make it more skin-friendly and, well, just plain better! Then my daughter asked me to write down my recipes so that she could inherit them. I was, needless to say, touched and flattered, and out of that grew my Skin-Friendly Recipes, which ended up being a key part of my Ageless Skin-Care program. I am pleased that I can now share with you my personal variations on classic recipes and newer ones as well in chapter 8. You have Sabrina, now thirteen and a very good skin-friendly cook, to thank for that! But as I said, I want you to do some experimenting of your own. Right now you may feel you simply don't have time for that, but once you get started, you'll realize that a little right-brained time in the kitchen will go a long way toward easing tension and tapping into your creative soul. So resist the urge to go to a fast-food drive-through to pick up dinner on your way home, and put down that phone if you were planning to call your local pizza parlor for a delivery.

Pearl: Don't go food shopping
when you're hungry.

Instead, keep a stock of healthy, fresh, frozen, and even some canned foods at home. I like to buy frozen vegetables since it is not always possible to get fresh seasonal vegetables. In fact even when fresh vegetables are available, I can't always get to the market every other day or so, and I don't like to have vegetables sit for too long in the refrigerator because they lose nutritional value. I find that when I buy frozen vegetables, I have more flexibility in what I can cook. I prefer to use fresh vegetables, but when foods are packaged to be sold frozen, they are picked fresh at peak or near-peak ripeness and then frozen. I call this "fresh frozen."

The process ensures that the produce stays essentially fresh until you use it. However, if you don't use the entire package, be sure to reseal frozen food properly in order to avoid freezer burn. But whether you use fresh or frozen ingredients, make a hobby and a habit out of inventive and skin-healthy cooking and get the whole family involved with the chopping and mincing. The process will go more quickly that way, and you'll have some wonderful together time with the people you love. Then you can all sit down to a meal you're proud of having made, and get the skin-boosting benefits of food that is both good and good for you.

NOURISHING YOUR SKIN WITH GOOD NUTRITION

Simply put, when skin-enhancing nutrients are ingested and absorbed into your bloodstream, they are delivered to your skin cells. And your skin needs all the nutritional help it can get because oxygen and blood carrying vital supplies of nutrients are rerouted away from your skin when your body perceives an emergency such as extreme cold or stress.

Your Skin Suffers When You're Cold

There is a plexus of blood vessels immediately under the dermis, and within the dermis, that is able to control large volumes of blood quickly. This is how the skin helps maintain a relatively constant temperature for the body, even under extreme circumstances. However, when you are exposed to extreme cold too suddenly, too often, or for too long, the skin pays a price in broken blood vessels and other changes as a result of its going into overdrive in order to protect your vital organs and help you survive. When you are very cold, your blood supply is concentrated inward to maintain and support your more vulnerable organs such as your brain and your heart. These organs are not able to tolerate fluctuations in their oxygen supply or temperature very well so the body prioritizes and sends the blood away from the skin to keep the "core" temperature as even and as close to normal as possible. We are designed to be able to lose a toe or a finger from frostbite and still survive, but we wouldn't do as well if we lost a part of the heart or brain! That's why your skin is the first organ to be deprived of nutrients and the last to receive them again when you are very cold or under a lot of stress.

Your Skin Suffers When You're Stressed

Stress, like extreme cold, is perceived by the body as an emergency situation and so blood is diverted either toward or away from your skin, both of which are bad for your skin. For example, you may turn beet red, or ghostly white, depending on the stressor—anger or fear, respectively. It may be that in primitive times, turning "white with fear" made us appear less visible, and turning "red with anger" showed that we were strong and ferocious so our adversaries would back off. Today, however, these inadvertent changes in the look of the skin most often do nothing but embarrass us by advertising to the world extreme emotions we'd rather keep to ourselves, especially if they turn out to be largely unwarranted. Obviously, you can't afford to consume anything less than optimal nutrition on a regular basis if you want to ensure that your skin will get through emergencies without "starving." Fortunately, your skin is a very resilient organ that has the capacity, and is designed, to tolerate these extremes to some extent, but at a price.

Your Skin Is Your Body's First Line of Defense

The other reason that your skin benefits from good nutrition is that your skin—your largest, most expandable organ and the one that is most exposed to the outside world—is responsible for protecting the rest of your body against damaging elements such as germs, ultraviolet rays, and pollution. These elements lead to inflammation, free-radical formation, and the potential for skin damage that goes with it. Eating foods containing nutrients called antioxidants that are capable of neutralizing free radicals boosts your skin's power to fend off damage and look younger longer. Free-radical damage is one of the main culprits involved in the rapid aging of the skin. Free radicals are highly unstable and reactive molecules that can damage all living cells. The most common way that free radicals are created is as by-products of the normal burning of fuel that occurs in every cell of the body every day. Your skin is also especially vulnerable to free-radical damage from external sources such as ultraviolet light from sunlight and pollutants that are all around you every day, especially if you live or work in a big city. Antioxidants have been getting so much attention lately that I think the entire concept can be overwhelming. I get questions every day like: Am I getting the right antioxidants? Do I need to take this specific patented one? Am I hurting my skin by not spending money on this or that product?

The answer is that antioxidants are truly very simple. They are a very large group of nutrients, often vitamins, or components of foods that we eat every day. They are so vital to survival that they are in just about everything we eat that is not overprocessed. The more we learn about specific antioxidants, the more we are able to isolate, stabilize, and concentrate them to make them more useful for skin-care products. Just because you are not eating a particular food or using a particular very expensive product does not in any way mean that you are depriving your body or your skin and ruining your health. There are a lot of overlapping ways that antioxidants work to help keep you at your healthy best.

NUTRIENTS YOU NEED FOR GOOD SKIN

In general, food that is good for your whole body is good for your skin. However, let's look at the list of nutrients that specifically make a positive difference in your skin.

Water-Soluble Antioxidants

These are not stored by your body in significant quantities. Most of the excess that you consume is eliminated through your urine. That's why you need to replenish your supply regularly, often on a daily basis. My Skin-Friendly Food Regimen will help you do exactly that.

Important Water-Soluble Nutrients

- Vitamin C
- Vitamin B complex

Fat-Soluble Antioxidants

These are stored in your body for longer periods than water-soluble antioxidants, which means that you don't need to replenish them every day. But it also means that you should not consume too much of them at one time. As a general rule, eating a balanced diet like my

Supplements

As a general rule, your best choice is to get as much as possible of your vitamins from food, not from supplements, although it is very difficult to get everything you need from the average diet especially if you are often rushed and resort to "fast food" that is overprocessed. An all-in-one supplement or a few separate specific supplements daily, these can be good insurance, but they won't take the place of eating right. Also, some ingredients inhibit the absorption of others and should be taken at different times when possible. For example, iron and calcium compete with each other for absorption so you should try not to take these supplements together. And there's no need for megadoses of water-soluble nutrients, vitamins B and C for example, because your body will use what it needs and get rid of the rest, storing very little at a time. In addition, don't be too concerned about the distinction between natural and synthetic supplements. Many products claim to be "all natural," as if the word "natural" means they are automatically safer, more potent, and better for you. This may be true in some cases. However, there are many instances in which synthetic vitamins can be as effective as, or even more effective than, their natural counterparts.

Here are some supplements you may want to consider adding to your diet for skin health or care to talk about with your physician.

- Calcium
- Folic acid
- Zinc
- Flaxseed or black currant oil
- DMAE and other fish oil supplements
- Magnesium
- Selenium
- Probiotic supplements such as acidophilus
- Coenzyme Q_{10}, an antioxidant
- Ellagic acid, an antioxidant precursor
- Alpha-lipoic acid, an antioxidant
- Carnosine, which helps prevent the binding of sugars to proteins, a negative process called glycation that often occurs when foods are cooked at very high temperatures
- Pycnogenol (available as a pill and in creams)
- Vitamin D

Skin-Friendly Food Regimen gives you enough of these nutrients. Again, you may wish to choose an all-in-one oral supplement, but avoid taking supplements that would give you extra doses of the fat-soluble nutrients. I have seen people taking supplements containing very large concentrations of both fat- and water-soluble vitamins and minerals. This can lead to toxicity and complications such as hair loss, kidney stones, and liver damage, depending on the ingredients ingested. Also, some nutrients can conflict with others. For example, large doses of the nutrient pantothenic acid have the potential to compete with biotin for intestinal and cellular uptake due to their similar structures.

Pearl: Most supplements should not be taken on an empty stomach. They will be excreted unless you also have food in your stomach to digest.

Important Fat-Soluble Nutrients

- Vitamin E
- Vitamin A
- Lycopene
- Coenzyme Q_{10}

Minerals

These are not antioxidants, but they boost the overall antioxidant ability of cells. They promote the production of important enzymes that give you more complete protection against oxidative damage. These are being added into skin-care products as well as to foods and vitamins with the goal of getting them to reach the skin where they are needed. You need only small amounts of these since their job is to boost and support other processes and so they don't get used up as quickly and are not needed in large amounts. We are seeing more and more research that shows not only the antiaging benefits of these nutrients, but also the anticancer benefits for many types of cancer. I would emphasize, however, that this is not a panacea. It is through regular screening that cancers are found and treated early. What I offer are suggestions to help you stay as healthy as possible, while expecting you to get your regular checkups as well.

Deficiencies of iron and copper can also adversely affect collagen and elastin production. Iron is found in whole grains and meat products. Copper deficiency is uncommon. However, if you take zinc supplements you are at a slightly higher risk of copper deficiency since these two nutrients compete for absorption.

Important minerals

- ᴄ Manganese
- ᴄ Copper
- ᴄ Zinc
- ᴄ Selenium

Phytochemicals

- ᴄ Isothiocyanates are a class of antioxidants found in foods such as watercress, horseradish, wasabi, mustard, and broccoli. Extracts of these are now also being used in some skin-care lines.
- ᴄ Ellagic acid can be supplied directly, or through the use of extracts of the foods that contain it, such as blueberries, cranberries, raspberries, green tea, grapes, wine, apples, pomegranates, walnuts, and pecans. All of these nutrients are powerful antioxidants because they neutralize potentially damaging free radicals in the entire cell. Cells have areas that respond to fat-soluble nutrients and other areas that respond to water-soluble nutrients. Nutrients that are both water- and fat-soluble are able to tackle both areas of a cell, giving you a complete defense against the skin-ravaging effects of free radicals.
- ᴄ Flavonoids are plant pigments that have antioxidant properties in addition to giving color to fruits, vegetables, and flowers. Some flavonoids are also good protection against allergies, viruses, inflammation, and even cancer. Research has shown

that two classes of flavonoids may be particularly good for your skin: proanthocyanidins, found in grapes, and polyphenols, found in green tea. The two classes, which include grape seed extract, green tea extract, and pine bark extract, are the most potent antioxidants yet identified. The best sources are pine bark, grape seed and skin, cranberries, green tea, blackberries, strawberries, cherries, red wine, red cabbage, and red apple skins. Pycnogenol is a standardized pine bark extract from the French maritime pine bark (*Pinus pinaster*) that is rich in proanthocyanidins. There is much research on this compound that validates its effects. It is known to slow the breakdown of collagen and elastin, thus improving the elasticity and resilience of the skin and therefore helping to maintain a youthful appearance. It is also known to protect against UVB damage. Research shows that not only is pycnogenol significantly more potent than vitamins C and E, it also helps recycle these vitamins and enhance their effect. It can be used topically or taken orally in the form of a supplement.

Fats

There are good fats and bad fats. Good fats are called monounsaturated or polyunsaturated, while bad fats are saturated and trans fats. Saturated fats are already listed on food labels, and the good news is that beginning in 2006 the amount of trans fats will also be required by law to be listed on labels. This has already prompted many companies to change the kinds of fats in their products. One of the best examples is Crisco, which just came out with a new and improved version that contains no trans fats. The sad fact is that the main purpose of the trans fats is to increase the shelf life of a product. That's all. Trans fats do not enhance flavor.

Here is a list of oils and fats you want to include in your diet. These not only help improve total cholesterol, but help reduce the "bad" cholesterol, LDL (low-density lipoprotein), and increase the "good" cholesterol, HDL (high-density lipoprotein). And when your cholesterol profile is healthy, your skin will look better!

- ᴄ Monounsaturated fats (These are the best ones to choose in general.)
  - Canola oil
  - Olive oil
  - Flaxseed oil
  - Most fish oils
- ᴄ Polyunsaturated fats
  - Safflower oil
  - Corn oil

Here is a list of oils and fats you want to minimize or avoid in your diet: The more saturated the fatty acid, the greater the detrimental effect on the total cholesterol and on the bad component called LDL. As always, your skin mirrors your overall health. There are also fatty deposits called xanthelasmas that can occur in the skin, often around the eyes, in some people who have very high cholesterol levels.

- ᴄ Saturated fats
  - Palmitic acid
  - Stearic acid
  - Myristic acid
  - Lauric acid
  - Partially hydrogenated oils (often found in cookies, other packaged desserts, and chips)
- ᴄ Trans fats (hydrogenated fats), which are made when hydrogen is added to vegetable oil to increase the shelf life of products such as vegetable shortening, crackers, and cookies.

Fiber

Fiber is very important for skin health because it promotes healthy, regular elimination of waste products. Constipation and hard stools lead to straining at each bowl movement, which can cause increased redness and broken blood vessels of the face over time if the condition is especially severe or chronic. You'll look more sallow and your face will show that you're not feeling your best. There are two types of fiber:

1. Soluble, found in fruits, vegetables, beans, and oats. These dissolve in water and help keep total cholesterol under control.
2. Insoluble, found in whole-grain foods such as wheat bran. These help us feel fuller and may help reduce the risk of colon cancer.

Both types of fiber are equally good for skin health, each in its own way.

KNOW YOUR NUTRIENTS

All of the nutrients you've learned about so far are important for good, glowing skin. However, certain nutrients are particularly instrumental in reversing the aging process in the skin. Let's have a look at these in detail.

Vitamin A

This is one of the most important vitamins for the skin. It is a fat-soluble family of vitamins, stored in the liver, with retinol being one of the most active forms. Vitamin A plays an important role in cell division. For the skin, this means that it helps the keratinocytes, or skin cells, mature in a normal healthy manner. The end result is skin that is smoother with even texture, which makes it a more effective barrier against infection. Vitamin A is also an important antioxidant, which is the reason it's an ingredient in many skin-care products.

Vitamin A deficiency in the skin causes dry skin that heals poorly and wrinkles more easily. The main sources of vitamin A are foods from animals, especially eggs, organ meats, and whole-milk dairy products. Since vitamin A is stored in fat, most foods that are high in vitamin A tend to be high in saturated fat and cholesterol. Some plants, such as carrots or broccoli, supply a precursor to vitamin A called beta-carotene that is converted to vitamin A by the body as needed. Other carotenoids commonly found in foods include lycopene, lutein, and zeaxanthin. They are not converted to vitamin A, but they are known to have health benefits such as anticancer and anti-inflammatory properties, and are being actively studied.

As with all things, too much of even a good thing can be problematic. While you can't get vitamin A toxicity from eating too much of the carotenoids, taking in too much vitamin A, either directly from high-dose supplements, or from eating large amounts of foods containing vitamin A, can lead to serious toxicity, which can in turn cause hair loss, problems with vision and bones, and other conditions you definitely want to avoid.

Good sources of beta-carotene and vitamin A include:

- Carrots (beta-carotene)
- Apricots (beta-carotene)
- Nectarines (beta-carotene)
- Plums (beta-carotene)
- Cantaloupe (beta-carotene)
- Fish oil
- Egg yolk
- Liver
- Milk

B-Complex Vitamins

The term B-complex usually refers to a group of vitamins that work together to support important metabolic functions of the body having to do with energy production. The group includes vitamins B_1 (thiamine), B_2 (riboflavin), B_3 (niacin), B_5 (pantothenate), B_6 (pyridoxine), B_{12} (cobalamin), biotin, and folate. True deficiencies of vitamins B_1 and B_2 have been shown to cause skin rashes, along with many other problems. Mild deficiencies are more subtle but still may lead to some degree of skin damage. Balancing the diet with B-complex supplements is a good idea but it does not help to go overboard. Your body will only use what it needs.

Vitamin B_{12} is essential for several cell functions. A deficiency of this vitamin can be especially damaging to the brain and to skin cells. Mild B_{12} deficiency often goes unnoticed since there are no obvious symptoms. Sometimes, people who show signs of depression may have a B_{12} deficiency as a contributing factor. B_{12} is the only vitamin that is found almost entirely in meat, poultry, fish, eggs, or dairy products, rather than plant sources. This means that people who are strict vegetarians may be at risk of vitamin B_{12} deficiency unless they take supplements.

Good sources of B-complex vitamins include:

- Tomatoes
- Meats
- Green peas
- Cranberries
- Yogurt
- Strawberries
- Sunflower seeds
- Squash

Folate is very important for rapidly dividing cells, especially skin cells. Vegetables such as green leafy vegetables and beans are the best sources of folate. The only animal source that is particularly rich in folate is liver. However, folate can be destroyed during cooking, so be sure to eat at least some of your vegetables fresh or only lightly cooked, to preserve this important nutrient.

Good sources of folate include:

- Lentils
- Lettuce
- Orange
- Okra
- Pinto beans, white beans
- Chickpeas
- Spinach
- Soybeans
- Liver

Vitamin C

Vitamin C is an especially important component of the anti-aging process because it is essential in the production of collagen. In some cases, vitamin C also acts as an antioxidant, and it has a synergistic effect with vitamins A and E as well as some fatty acids to enhance their antioxidant abilities. When vitamin C binds to a fatty acid called palmitic acid, through a process called esterification, the result is a fat-soluble form of vitamin C that functions as an effective antioxidant. This is sold commercially as vitamin C ester and should not be confused with a different commercially available product called ester-C. Deficiency of vitamin C leads to a disease called scurvy, first discovered in sailors who did not get adequate vitamin C on long voyages. The signs are poor wound healing, bumps of curled hair on the arms and legs, easy bruising, bleeding gums, loose teeth, joint pain, and more. Vitamn C is sensitive to cooking, so it is best obtained from raw fruits and vegetables. Vitamin C is a water-soluble vitamin that is also stored in the liver. The recommended daily allowance of vitamin C for women is 75 mg.

Good sources of vitamin C include:

- Citrus fruits such as limes, oranges, grapefruit
- Other fruit: watermelon, apricots, mangoes, peaches, pears, papaya, pumpkin, cantaloupe, berries
- Bell peppers
- Barley
- Navy beans
- Broccoli
- Brussels sprouts
- Cucumber
- Green peas
- Tomatoes
- Potatoes

Vitamin E (Tocopherol)

Vitamin E is one of the most significant antioxidants found in the human body when it comes to skin health and rejuvenation. It is recommended both in topical and oral forms for everything from wound healing to improvement of stretch marks as well as a very long list of antiaging and anticancer roles. A fat-soluble vitamin, it plays an important part in protecting the fatty lining of the cells called cell membranes from free radical damage. These membranes are otherwise left very susceptible to this type of damage. Since all vitamins are vital for life, hence the name, it makes sense that the diet needs a source of vitamin E in order for us to survive. However, because it is fat soluble, a small amount goes a long way. The body uses what it needs and then stores the rest. It is uncommon to see vitamin E deficiency in most diets. As long as you're eating a balanced diet, you should be getting enough vitamin E. It is a good additive to look for in topical skin preparations, though.

Good sources of vitamin E include:

- Sunflower seeds
- Tomatoes
- Turnip greens
- Peaches
- Papaya
- Spinach
- Pumpkin

Coenzyme Q$_{10}$

Coenzyme Q$_{10}$ (CoQ$_{10}$) is another very important ingredient that is getting a lot of attention lately, both in skin-care products and as a supplement, because of its skin-enhancing antioxidant properties. It is also called ubiquinone, since it is found in such a wide variety of foods and because it is produced by every cell in the body. This makes it ubiquitous, hence the name ubiquinone. A fat-soluble vitamin like compound, it is an antioxidant and a significant coenzyme in several critical pathways of energy production of the body. The ability of the body to produce CoQ$_{10}$ decreases over time and among patients on certain types of medicine, such as certain cholesterol-lowering drugs. It is found in small amounts in almost every food we eat.

Cysteine and Methionine

Cysteine and methionine are related sulfur-containing amino acids. Amino acids are the building blocks of proteins. These amino acids are special since they also work as antioxidants and assist in controlling the absorption of toxic and skin-spoiling heavy metals such as lead. Cysteine is also a component of glutathione, which is the primary water-soluble antioxidant inside cells. While most of the amino acids can be produced by our bodies, methionine is an exception to that rule, meaning we have to get it from our diet. Foods containing these nutrients include soybeans and other foods high in protein such as fish, chicken, beef, liver, eggs, and cheese. Overall, cysteine and methionine contribute to good skin health because they are potent antioxidants and therefore are enemies of the free radicals that can damage your skin.

Alpha-Lipoic Acid

Alpha-lipoic acid plays an important role in energy production. It helps the cell generate energy from carbohydrates. It is also an antioxidant in its own right and it helps extend the life of other antioxidants such as vitamins C and E and glutathione. The body can make some alpha-lipoic acid but cannot make enough to meet increased need during periods of stress or in cases of chronic illness. As we've already noted, alpha-lipoic acid is both water and fat soluble, and it is one of the more useful antioxidants since it protects against most types of free radicals. It also has many other important functions, such as chelating (neutralizing) damaging metals, which makes this an ingredient you want to be sure you get enough of in your diet. This is why some of the newer diet plans single out lipoic acid among all the antioxidants out there. The best source of alpha-lipoic acid is red meat.

DR. DAY'S OWN MIDLIFE NUTRITION MAKEOVER

After my fortieth birthday, I learned the hard way that my skin and body are less forgiving of indulgences than they were before forty. Without much effort, since I considered myself still young but wiser, I modified my eating habits for the better. Here are my nutrition makeover secrets:

Pearl: The next time you think about "cheating," take your urge out of the closet. Celebrate it and take control of it. Put your treat on a nice plate and enjoy every bite.

Forget the Fries

I gave up French fries except for a few—and I mean a few—here and there if I decide that they're worth it. For the most part, fries are greasy, empty calories that leave you too full to eat the nutritious food that will give your skin a healthy glow.

Hold the Desserts

I still enjoy a piece of birthday cake or wedding cake or other special occasion treats, but on a daily basis I gave up desserts. Again, sweets are usually a deceivingly enticing combination of unhealthy fats and simple sugars that do nothing for my skin or my health. I have learned to enjoy, with passion, foods that are beautiful and colorful and healthful, so I can now appreciate an attractive, well-presented dessert as a work of art, but I have no desire to eat it.

Start the Day with a Lemon Elixir

Every morning, I enjoy a glass of water laced with the juice of half a fresh lemon. This is a delicious, no-calorie way to begin hydrating my skin immediately after I wake up.

Have Fruit for Breakfast

I eat a generous portion of select fresh fruit, most often berries or grapefuit, in the morning in order to get a head start on the antioxidants that will take care of skin-damaging free radicals.

Have a Hearty Lunch

I treat myself to a wonderful, satisfying, healthful lunch. That way, I'm not starving by dinnertime, and I'm not tempted to gulp down more food than I really need or grab unhealthy food rather than cook nutritious, skin-friendly food.

Eat a Light Dinner

I eat less at dinner than I do at lunch. After all, I keep burning calories during the hours that I'm active after lunch, but after dinner I just go to bed. My body doesn't really need a huge meal at dinner.

Don't Eat After Dinner

I make sure that dinner is over before my personal eating deadline of 8 P.M. I came up with this time because I typically go to bed at about 10 P.M. This gives me time to digest my dinner, and it assures that I won't give in to an urge snack before bed even though I don't need more food. You can adjust this rule to suit your own schedule. Just commit to an eating deadline that is about two hours before your regular bedtime.

WEIGHT-LOSS BONUS

If you follow my guidelines above, your skin will benefit immensely. In addition, as a wonderful bonus, any extra pounds you've wanted

> *Pearl:* The best kind of weight loss is unintentional because you're eating right and enjoying it.

to lose will seem to "fall off" as they did for me. Losing weight truly does not have to be a struggle. Mind-set is a very large part of success. Every time I would try to diet or even consciously think about restricting my caloric intake, I would gain a pound or two. Even the idea of being deprived was very scary. It made me feel as though I were constantly starving and I would even almost panic about being hungry. However, once I looked at the situation from the point of view that I was going to focus on other areas of my life and not dwell on what I could or could not eat, I found that I was able to eat what I liked, which was mostly food that was healthy and satisfying. The weight came off so much more easily and I felt great. Here's how you can have the same results.

Don't Think of Dieting as Deprivation

Forget right now and forever the idea that "going on a diet" is a temporary act of deprivation during which time just about everything that tastes good is forbidden. Eating should be a joy and a celebration, not a battle about what you can have and how many calories you can get away with. You should revel in every bite, savor every morsel, and cherish every meal. This means, don't sit in front of the TV, read, or ignore your food while you are eating. I remember so many times, sitting on the couch with a full bowl of something and then looking down and seeing it empty. There was no one else there but me, but I had very little recollection of eating the food or of how it tasted. I felt full, but not satisfied. Now I turn off the TV and I give my meal all the attention it deserves. I end up feeling full and satisfied. What a difference focusing on your meal makes!

Break Out of the Yo-yo Dieting Cycle

One of the worst things you can do for your skin in terms of diet is the yo-yo, up-and-down syndrome that stresses the skin. Yet that is exactly what happens if you think of dieting as a short-term, crash-it-off concept. The rapid weight loss of the down cycle adds to the jowls and wrinkles that we are trying so hard to avoid. I lost nearly sixty pounds without ever using the word "diet." And I've had no trouble keeping the weight off for many years. As a matter of fact, eliminating the concept of going on a diet was the first step to getting me back on the right path. This approach works for my patients, and it will work for you as well. My Skin-Friendly Food Regimen is nutritionally correct, based on solid medical research, and it's designed to bring you a lifetime of pleasurable eating that will give your skin the glow of optimal health.

Leave the Last Bite on Your Plate

If you finish everything on your plate, and even scrape it clean with bread to get every last drop, you are sending a message to your brain that there was not enough food. You are letting the portion dictate how hungry you are. If you make a decision that you are done before the portion is finished, you send a very strong message to your mind and through it to your stomach that you have had enough and you couldn't eat another bite. This strategy gives you control over how much is enough. It makes a dramatic difference in how you look at food, and your level of satisfaction will increase significantly. The only foods that I finish to the last drop are my berries and fruits.

Pearl: Losing weight slowly—no more than one to two pounds per week—not only helps you keep the weight off but also avoid saggy jowls and a "turkey wattle" neck from loose skin. Just be sure to exercise your face, along with your body, while you're paring off pounds. That way, your face will be as firm as possible forever!

Challenge Your Metabolism

Another key aspect of my meal plan is that you will challenge your metabolism by varying the number of calories you eat overall—more on some days, less on others—while increasing your exercise level. This will allow you to lose weight, become toned, and get your metabolism working to your advantage. If you lower the number of calories you take in and don't challenge your metabolism, your metabolic rate will slow down and you will get stuck in your weight loss after a certain point. Your body will be working against you. If you vary your diet so that you get more calories once in a while, your metabolism will speed up to meet the need of burning the extra calories without your gaining any weight. Then over the next few days when you eat less again, your metabolism will still be higher so your body will burn fat to meet the energy needs of the higher metabolic rate.

Pearl: It is easier not to gain weight than it is to lose it.

Get Moving

If you add in exercise, you will maintain a higher metabolic rate, which will expedite the process even further. You'll be getting the skin-firming benefits of exercise right along with your Skin Friendly Food Regimen. I'll tell you more about what exercise can do for your skin when we get to step 4.

I'm hoping that by now you just can't wait to start cooking up some delicious, nutritious, skin-friendly food using the recipes and meal plans in the following chapter, and some of your own as well. But before you do, I want to remind you one more time that while proper nutrition can definitely play a big role in staving off wrinkles and other signs of skin aging, eating right is only one of the key elements in my Ageless Skin-Care program. You need to continue to incorporate into your life all that you have learned so far in this book. Especially important—and I simply cannot say this to you often enough—is to limit sun exposure and use sunblock every day, all year long.

Okay, the lecture is over! Now you're ready to learn about my Ageless Skin Meal Plan complete with irresistible recipes for skin-friendly dishes.

Pearl: Snacking intermittently during the day on healthy food such as certain fruits and vegetables helps you stave off hunger pangs that can cause you to grab an unhealthy snack such as a candy bar or a slice of pizza. Snacking also helps you control portions of your meals and meal choices.

8

Skin–Friendly Food

If you begin my Skin-Friendly Meal Plan right now during step 3 of my Ageless Skin-Care program, you'll see a definite difference in the look of your skin by the end of one week. And as the weeks go by, your skin will look even younger. As a bonus, you'll be paring off any pounds you may need to lose. You'll also be feeling energetic and very good about yourself. As if that weren't enough, you'll be enjoying what you eat more than you ever have before!

A SKIN-FRIENDLY MEAL PLAN

What follows is a five-day plan designed to get your skin glowing in a hurry. Naturally, I recommend following a variation of this plan from now on. I've given you recipes for some of the skin-friendly dishes in the meal plan, plus extra recipes to keep you going after the five days are up.

Every day you should have two snacks, one between breakfast and lunch and one between lunch and dinner. Choose from the following list of skin-friendly snacks:

- A bowl of strawberries, raspberries, blueberries, or blackberries, alone or with Honey Dipping Sauce (see page 211). Do not have the Honey Dipping Sauce more than two times per week.
- A bunch of grapes. Eat the seeds as well. They are full of antioxidants and fiber.
- A couple of plums or apricots, alone or with Honey Dipping Sauce
- Vegetable crudités with homemade or low-fat hummus or avocado dip
- A small handful of unsalted nuts or seeds
- A large slice of melon or pineapple, alone or with Honey Dipping Sauce
- A banana, alone or with peanut butter-honey spread (see page 211)
- Fruit smoothie

Day 1

Breakfast: 8 oz. plain or vanilla nonfat yogurt; one cup of fresh fruit salad

Lunch: Open-faced Grilled Chicken Sandwich and Grilled Vegetables (page 198); tangerine or small fruit of your choice

Dinner: Herbed Salmon (page 201), green salad, string beans with a light garlic sauce

Pearl: If you try hard enough for long
enough, you will get there—and, oh, does
it feel good when you do!

Day 2

Breakfast: Oatmeal/Whole-Wheat Pancakes (page 189); a
small bowl of fresh fruit. (As you make your own meal
plans in the weeks that follow, opt for this menu option not
more than two or three times per week. Choose the other
breakfasts on this list for the rest of the days.)

Lunch: Grilled Vegetable Bruschetta (page 199); Tossed
Baby Greens and Tomato salad (page 192)

Dinner: Chicken with Vegetable Stir-fry (page 202);
Arugula Salad (page 193)

Day 3

Breakfast: Bowl of oatmeal made with low-fat or fat-free
milk or soy milk. If you are lactose intolerant, choose lac-
tose-reduced or lactose-free milk. Sprinkle your oatmeal
with cinnamon, a few raisins, and toasted almonds.

Lunch: Tuna Salad (page 193); Vegetable Soup (page 191)

Dinner: Garlic Chicken with Zucchini and Wild Rice
(page 202), Cucumber and Tomato Salad (page 194)

Day 4

Breakfast: Scrambled Eggs with Herbs (page 190) or a vegetable omelet; a bowl of fresh fruit salad. (As you make you own meal plans in the weeks that follow, opt for this menu not more than two or three times per week.) Choose other breakfasts on this list for the rest of the days.

Lunch: Chicken Salad (page 195)

Dinner: Quick Salmon Steak with Teriyaki Sauce (page 203); Spinach Salad with Pomegranate (page 195)

Day 5

Breakfast: Plate of fresh fruit such as peaches, strawberries, kiwi, blueberries, raspberries (if you choose to add banana use ½ medium-sized banana; if you can only get canned fruit, rinse off the juice); 1 to 2 tablespoons of toasted nuts, such as almonds, hazelnuts, or cashews

Lunch: Goat Cheese Salad (page 196)

Dinner: Tabouleh Salad with Diced Chicken (page 197)

RECIPES

Following are recipes for some meals that I recommend be part of your meal plans. I have created these recipes from years of cooking and experimenting. I have always loved to cook and when I set my kitchen up in a way that was comfortable and had a smooth flow in terms of the way bowls, pots, pans, and ingredients were organized, I found that I loved it even more. The kitchen is such a powerful place. It is full of warmth and nourishment. Make your kitchen a place where you want to spend time putting together easy, healthy recipes for beautiful skin.

Breakfasts

Oatmeal/Whole-Wheat Pancakes
Makes 2 servings

3 egg whites
¼ cup plain old-fashioned whole-oat oatmeal
½ cup whole-wheat flour
1 teaspoon baking powder
Dash of salt
½ teaspoon cinnamon
¼ teaspoon nutmeg
⅓ cup low-fat milk
1 teaspoon vanilla extract

Beat the egg whites until stiff. Set aside.

In a mixing bowl, combine the oatmeal, flour, baking powder, salt, cinnamon, and nutmeg and mix until evenly combined. Add the milk and vanilla and blend for one minute on high speed. Fold the egg whites into the batter until just blended.

Place 2 tablespoons of batter onto a hot pan sprayed with nonstick spray. When you see bubbles forming on top of the pancake, it is ready to be flipped over.

Transfer to a serving plate.

Scrambled Eggs with Herbs
Makes 1 serving

1 whole egg
1 egg white
¼ teaspoon parsley
¼ teaspoon basil
¼ teaspoon pepper

In a small mixing bowl, beat the egg and egg white until well blended and frothy. Add the herbs and mix until well blended.

Coat a pan with nonstick spray and add the egg mixture. Scramble until well done.

Transfer to a serving plate. Top with a few sprigs of fresh parsley. Serve with a few slices of fresh orange.

Fruit-Filled Melon
Makes 2 servings

½ cantaloupe
½ orange, peeled and sectioned
½ small apple, coarsely chopped
¼ cup blueberries
¼ cup raspberries
¼ cup strawberries
1 cup low-fat vanilla yogurt, stirred until creamy

Using a melon scoop, scoop out all of the cantaloupe flesh. Alternatively, cut out all of the flesh into scoops. Set the shell aside.

In a mixing bowl, combine all of the fruit, then transfer the fruit mixture to the shelled melon for serving. Pour the yogurt over the fruit.

Soups

Vegetable Soup

You can divide the soup you don't eat into portions and freeze in freezer bags/containers and have it on another day.

Makes 2 servings

1 teaspoon canola oil

1 to 2 onions, chopped

4 cloves garlic, chopped

2 stalks celery, chopped

3 cups water (or if you have chicken stock, you can use
   that instead of the water, and then you don't need the
   bouillon cube)

1 chicken or vegetable low-salt bouillon cube

2 bay leaves

1 eight-ounce can crushed tomatoes

2 small ripe tomatoes, diced

1 small carrot, chopped

In a saucepan, sauté the onions, garlic, and celery in oil until almost brown. Add water, bay leaves, bouillon cube (if using), tomatoes, and carrots. Bring to a boil, then place on low heat and simmer for 2 to 3 hours.

Serve topped with fresh ground pepper.

Green Split Pea Soup

Slow-cook this recipe on a weekend or when you have time. You can freeze the part you don't use for another time.

Makes 4 servings

1 16-ounce (1 pound) bag green split peas
1 medium onion, minced
2 cloves garlic, minced
1 large shallot, minced
1 cup low-sodium chicken broth
8 fresh ripe tomatoes, puréed, plus ½ cup water; or 1 28-ounce
   can crushed tomatoes
1 tablespoon olive oil

Soak the peas in warm water for 1 to 2 hours, or overnight. Sauté the onions, garlic, and shallot in oil until softened but not yet brown. Add the chicken broth. You can add more or less broth to make it thinner or thicker as you like (I prefer it soupier but my family likes it thicker and more like a stew). Add the peas. Heat until boiling, then cover and simmer for 2 to 3 hours, until the peas are soft. Add the tomatoes and cook for 20 to 30 minutes more. Serve hot.

Salads

Tossed Baby Greens and Tomato Salad
Makes 1 serving

1 cup baby greens
1 medium tomato, chopped

Dressing
1 teaspoon extra-virgin olive oil
About 1 teaspoon balsamic vinegar or lemon juice to taste
Dash of salt
Pepper to taste

In a serving bowl, mix the greens and tomato. In a small bowl, combine the dressing ingredients. Add to the salad and toss.

Arugula Salad
Makes 1 serving

1 cup chopped arugula
⅓ cup shredded radicchio
½ teaspoon extra-virgin olive oil
2 tablespoons lemon juice (optional)
Dash of salt
Fresh ground pepper to taste

Mix the argula and radicchio in a salad bowl. Toss with the olive oil and lemon juice, if using. Add salt and pepper to taste.

Tuna Salad
Makes 2 servings

1 7-ounce can albacore tuna in water, rinsed and drained
1 shallot, chopped
1 red bell pepper, chopped
½ stalk celery, chopped
1 small lemon, peeled and sliced
1 leaf of romaine or Boston lettuce

Dressing
1 tablespoon extra-virgin olive oil
¼ cup lemon juice
2 tablespoons fresh, chopped, or dried dill
Salt, fresh ground pepper to taste

To make the salad, combine the tuna, shallot, pepper, and celery in a bowl.

To make the dressing, combine all of the ingredients in a small bowl. Set aside.

Place the lettuce leaf on a serving plate with lemon slices as a border. Arrange the tuna mixture on top of the lettuce leaf and sprinkle the dressing over the top.

Cucumber and Tomato Salad

Makes 2 servings

1 cucumber, peeled and diced
2 medium tomatoes, diced
1 small red onion, diced

Dressing
1 teaspoon extra-virgin olive oil
¼ cup lemon juice or vinegar (you can add more or less to taste)
Dash of salt

Toss the vegetables in a bowl. In a separate bowl, combine the dressing ingredients. Toss the dressing in with the vegetables. Transfer to a serving plate. Top with fresh ground pepper to taste.

Chicken Salad

Makes 1 serving

½ cup finely chopped cooked chicken
1 stalk celery, chopped
1 green onion, sliced
1 tablespoon lemon juice
Dash of pepper
2 hard-boiled egg whites
2 tablespoons low-fat mayonnaise or mayonnaise substitute
2 tablespoons green pepper, chopped
½ teaspoon mustard
1 tomato, cut in half, center scooped out

In a mixing bowl, combine the chicken, celery, onion, lemon juice, and pepper. Stir in the egg whites, mayonnaise, green pepper, and mustard. Place salad mixture in the tomato halves.

If you make the chicken salad in advance, store the mixed ingredients in the refrigerator and place inside the tomato just before you're ready to serve.

Alternatively, you could serve the salad on a bed of romaine or baby green lettuce.

Spinach Salad with Pomegranate

Makes 2 servings

2 cups fresh spinach, torn into bite-size pieces
1 small tomato, quartered
2 tablespoons pomegranate seeds

Dressing
1 tablespoon lemon juice
½ teaspoon flaxseed oil
½ teaspoon extra-virgin olive oil
Pepper to taste

Mix the salad ingredients in a serving bowl. Set aside.

To make the dressing, combine the ingredients in a small cup until well mixed. Toss with the salad. Transfer to serving plate.

Goat Cheese Salad

Makes 2 servings

½ head Boston lettuce, torn into bite-size pieces
½ head radicchio, shredded
2 slices goat cheese about ¼ inch thick each

Dressing
½ small shallot, minced
1 small clove garlic, minced (or ¼ teaspoon minced garlic from a jar)
1 tablespoon lemon juice
2 teaspoons Dijon mustard

To make the dressing, combine the ingredients in a small cup and mix well. Set aside. Toss the lettuce and radicchio with the dressing. Pile the lettuce on each serving plate. Place a slice of goat cheese over each salad. Add fresh ground pepper to taste.

Tabouleh Salad with Diced Chicken

To save time, you can use a tabouleh mix instead. Just follow the instructions on the box and add the chicken and dressing when the tabouleh is ready.

Makes 4 servings

½ cup bulgur, cooked
¼ cup diced sweet red pepper
¼ cup diced green pepper
3 tablespoons chopped scallion
3 tablespoons chopped parsley
¼ cup diced, seeded plum tomatoes
1 medium cucumber, seeds removed, coarsely chopped
2 chicken breasts, grilled and diced
1 large romaine lettuce leaf

Dressing
⅛ cup extra-virgin olive oil
¼ cup lemon juice
1 teaspoon dried mint
¼ teaspoon minced garlic
Dash of salt
Pepper to taste

To prepare the dressing, combine all ingredients in a small bowl. Set aside.

Combine the tabouleh ingredients in a large bowl. Add the chicken. Mix in the dressing. Place a lettuce leaf on a serving plate, and spoon the mixture over the lettuce leaf.

Chicken Caesar My Way
Makes 1 serving

½ head romaine lettuce, chilled and cut or torn into bite-size pieces
1 4-ounce chicken breast, grilled and cut into strips
2 hard-boiled egg whites, chopped or diced
½ hard-boiled egg yolk, crumbled
1 teaspoon crumbled blue cheese
½ teaspoon grated Parmesan cheese

Dressing
½ teaspoon extra-virgin olive oil
1 garlic clove, minced
⅛ cup lemon juice (I like more, you may opt to use less)
Tabasco sauce to taste
Dash of salt
¼ teaspoon dry mustard

To make the dressing, combine the ingredients and stir vigorously to blend. Set aside.

In a large bowl, place the chilled romaine lettuce. Add the dressing and toss.

Transfer to a serving plate. Place the chicken strips and the egg over the top. Sprinkle the cheeses over salad.

Sandwiches

Open-faced Grilled Chicken Sandwich and Grilled Vegetables
Makes 2 servings

2 slices red onion
¼ cup chopped red bell pepper

1 tablespoon finely chopped garlic or roasted garlic

¾ cup chopped or shredded fresh spinach

¼ teaspoon turmeric

2 tablespoons dry white wine

½ cup sliced mushrooms

Whole-wheat or whole-grain roll, toasted, halved crosswise

1 boneless breast of chicken, grilled, cut into strips

1 tablespoon fresh chopped parsley or parsley flakes

Coat a medium skillet with nonstick spray and sauté the onion, pepper, garlic, spinach, and turmeric until the vegetables are tender. Stir in the wine. Add the mushrooms. Cover and cook about 4 minutes, until the mushrooms are just tender. Place a half roll each on 2 serving plates. Layer the strips of chicken on the roll halves, followed by the vegetable mixture. Top with a sprinkle of parsley and pepper to taste.

Grilled Vegetable Bruschetta

Makes 1 serving

½ red bell pepper, grilled, chopped

½ yellow bell pepper, grilled, chopped

½ small onion, grilled, chopped

2 plum tomatoes, diced

½ teaspoon garlic, minced

1 large slice of whole-grain bread, toasted

1 teaspoon extra-virgin olive oil

In a small bowl, combine the vegetables. Place toast on a serving plate. Spread the vegetables over the toast. Drizzle the olive oil over vegetables.

Tuna Salad on Rye
Makes 2 servings

1 7-ounce can tuna in water
1 tablespoon low-fat mayonnaise
1 teaspoon lemon juice
½ stalk celery, chopped
4 leaves baby greens
2 slices rye bread, lightly toasted and cut into 4 squares each

In a small mixing bowl combine the tuna, mayo, lemon juice, and celery until evenly mixed. Place the green leaves over each side of the toast. Add the tuna over the greens. You can place a slice of lettuce and toast on top or eat as an open-faced sandwich.

Cucumber and Cilantro Sandwich
Makes 1 serving

1 cup fresh cilantro leaves
½ cup fresh mint leaves
1 fresh jalapeño pepper, seeded
1 clove garlic
1 to 2 tablespoons lime juice
2 slices whole-wheat bread, lightly toasted
1-ounce slice low-fat provolone cheese, cut into
    ¼ inch-thick strips
1 medium cucumber, thinly sliced (about ½ cup)

In a food processor (or by hand) finely chop the cilantro, mint, jalapeño pepper, and garlic with the lime juice. On a serving plate, place 1 bread slice. Top with half of the slices of cheese. Place the cucumber slices over the cheese. Add the cilantro mixture, followed by remaining cheese and the other bread slice. Cut the sandwich in half.

Entrées

Herbed Salmon
Makes 2 servings

2 6-ounce fresh or frozen skinless wild Alaskan King salmon
    fillets, ¾-inch thick, rinsed and patted dry
1 fresh lemon, cut in half
¼ cup coarsely chopped fresh oregano
¼ cup coarsely chopped fresh cilantro
¼ cup coarsely chopped almonds
1 green onion, chopped into small pieces
2 cloves garlic, minced
2 teaspoons lemon juice
⅛ teaspoon pepper

Rub each side of the salmon with a lemon half, squeezing the lemon gently as you go to release the juice. Set aside.

In a heavy zip storage bag, combine the oregano, cilantro, chopped almonds, and pepper. Put the fillets in the bag and shake to coat the fish.

Cook the salmon with the garlic and lemon juice on a preheated grill (I really love my countertop nonstick electric grill; it also has interchangeable griddle tops for cooking eggs and pancakes) for 6 to 8 minutes, or until the salmon just begins to flake easily with a fork, or broil for about 2 minutes on each side. Do not overcook. Cut each salmon piece in half. Transfer to a serving plate. Top with a sprinkle of fresh or dried parsley and fresh ground pepper to taste.

Chicken with Vegetable Stir-fry
Makes 1 serving

½ teaspoon canola oil

1 4-ounce chicken breast, cubed

¼ teaspoon ginger, finely chopped; or ½ teaspoon ginger powder

1 small onion, chopped

1 cup frozen mixed vegetables containing broccoli, green beans,
    and red/yellow peppers, thawed to room temperature

1 tablespoon low-sodium soy sauce

1 teaspoon water

½ teaspoon sesame oil

Heat canola oil in a wok or saucepan. Add the chicken and cook until barely pink. Add the onion and ginger. Cook until lightly browned. Add the vegetables, soy sauce, water, and sesame oil. Stir until the chicken is completely cooked. Do not overcook vegetables. Serve with ½ cup wild rice.

Garlic Chicken with Zucchini and Wild Rice
Makes 1 serving

1 green onion, sliced

1 teaspoon canola oil

1 teaspoon low-sodium soy sauce

2 teaspoons dry white wine

3 cloves garlic, chopped, or 3 tablespoons minced garlic

¼ cup water

1 medium zucchini, thinly sliced

½ cup sliced mushrooms

1 boneless, skinless chicken breast sliced thin

1 teaspoon paprika

½ cup cooked brown or wild rice
ground black pepper

Sauté the onion in the canola oil until browned. Add the soy sauce, white wine, garlic, and water. Add the zucchini. Once zucchini appears slightly softened, add mushrooms, cook for 2 to 3 minutes more. Set aside.

Sprinkle the chicken with paprika and grill until tender. Make sure the chicken is not pink before removing it from grill.

Place ½ cup rice on serving plate. Place the chicken over the rice. Layer the zucchini mix over the chicken. Top with coarsely ground pepper.

Quick Salmon Steak with Teriyaki Sauce
Makes 1 serving

1 4-ounce salmon steak
2 tablespoons low-sodium teriyaki sauce

Baste the salmon with low-sodium teriyaki sauce. Grill until flaky. Serve topped with a fresh parsley sprig.

Pan-Seared Tilapia
Makes 1 serving

1 4-ounce tilapia fillet
¼ cup coarsely chopped almonds
¼ teaspoon dried basil
¼ teaspoon pepper

Rinse the fish and pat dry. In a heavy-duty zip-top bag, mix the almonds, basil, and pepper. Place the fish in the bag and gently turn to coat the fish. Cook in a nonstick skillet until flaky. Transfer to a serving plate. Add fresh ground pepper to taste.

Grilled Salmon Cubes and Onion

Makes 1 serving

Marinade
¼ cup lemon juice
1 teaspoon paprika
Dash of salt

1 4-ounce salmon steak, cubed
1 small green onion, chopped
2 cloves garlic, minced

To make the marinade, combine the lemon juice, paprika, and salt in a large covered bowl. Marinate the salmon steaks in the mixture for at least a half hour (overnight is better).

Lightly coat a pan with nonstick cooking spray. Sauté the onion and garlic until slightly tender. Add the salmon cubes and continue to sauté until just cooked. Transfer to serving plate. Serve with broccoli rabe or creamed spinach.

Pan-Roasted Chicken Breasts

Makes 2 servings

Marinade
½ cup lemon juice
1 tablespoon kosher salt (or ½ tablespoon table salt)
1 small onion, coarsely chopped
1 shallot, coarsely chopped

2 boneless, skinless chicken breast fillets (slice the breasts in half, but do not completely separate, so they become thinner but remain as one piece)

1 teaspoon paprika

1 tablespoon canola or safflower oil

Sauce

1 large shallot, minced

½ cup low-sodium chicken broth

¼ cup dry red wine

¼ cup red wine vinegar

1 bay leaf

Mix marinade ingredients in an airtight sealable container. Place the chicken in the marinade and turn to coat evenly. Place in refrigerator to marinate for at least a half hour (overnight is better).

Remove the chicken from the marinade and sprinkle both sides with paprika. Heat the oil in a heavy-bottomed ovenproof skillet. Gently place the chicken in the hot oil for about 5 minutes on each side or until it turns a golden brown. Set aside while you make the sauce.

To make the sauce, in the same skillet, sauté the shallot. Add the chicken broth, wine, vinegar, and bay leaf. Stir constantly over high flame to thicken and reduce mixture to about ½ cup. Pour over the chicken. Serve with a side of Creamed Spinach (see page 210).

Roasted Cod with Broccoli and Sweet Peppers
Makes 2 servings

1 yellow bell pepper, cut into 1-inch-wide strips

1 red bell pepper, cut into 1-inch-wide strips

1 stalk broccoli with stem, chopped

4 cloves garlic, chopped

1 tablespoon olive oil

½ pound cod fillets with skin, cut into 2 pieces

1 sprig fresh rosemary

4 lemon wedges

Preheat oven to 450°F.

In a skillet, sauté or grill the peppers, broccoli, and garlic until tender. Transfer the peppers and broccoli to a cutting board and finely chop. Rinse the cod fillets and pat dry with paper towels. Sprinkle salt and pepper on both sides of each fillet. Heat the oil in a large oven-proof nonstick skillet over medium-high heat. Add the cod, skin-side down, and cook 2 to 3 minutes, until skin is crisp and golden brown. Arrange the rosemary on top of the fish. Transfer the skillet to the oven and roast 3 minutes. Turn the fish; roast 3 minutes more, until fish is opaque and cooked through. Transfer to a serving plate and spoon the pepper/broccoli/garlic mixture evenly on top of each fillet and serve with side of Arugula Salad (page 193).

Cold Grilled Sweet Peppers with Tofu
Makes 1 serving

¼ cup low-sodium chicken broth

1 tablespoon low-sodium soy sauce

½ tablespoon grated ginger

1 teaspoon safflower oil

2 cloves garlic, minced

1 stalk fresh broccoli, chopped into bite-size pieces

1 onion, chopped

½ cup frozen chopped spinach, thawed to room temperature

1 medium sweet red pepper, cut into thin strips

4 ounces extra-firm tofu, drained and cut into ½-inch cubes

In a mixing bowl, combine the chicken broth, soy sauce, and ginger. Set aside.

Stir-fry the garlic in hot oil until barely brown. Add the broccoli, onion, spinach, and sweet pepper and stir-fry until just tender. Add the chicken broth mixture. Stir and add the tofu. Cover and cook for about 5 minutes, or until the tofu is hot. Refrigerate and serve cold over a bed of green lettuce or serve hot over ½ cup wild rice.

Side Dishes

String Beans with Garlic Sauce
Makes 2 servings

1 cup string beans
2 cloves garlic, minced
½ teaspoon olive oil
1 teaspoon lemon juice

Lightly steam the string beans so they remain crunchy and bright green. In a pan, sauté the garlic in olive oil and lemon juice until the garlic is barely brown. Transfer the string beans to a serving plate and spoon the garlic sauce over them.

Spinach and Yogurt

This is one of my favorites. It is a Middle Eastern recipe that is full of calcium and vitamin C and contains very little fat. I serve it as a side dish with grilled chicken and wild rice, or just as a snack.

1 8-ounce package frozen chopped spinach, thawed
1 32-ounce container fat-free plain yogurt

1 shallot, chopped
1 clove garlic, chopped
Dash of salt
Pepper to taste

Steam the spinach until bright green and soft. Combine the yogurt, spinach, shallot, and garlic in a mixing bowl. Mix until well blended. Add salt and pepper to taste.

Baked Potato with Guacamole Dip

Makes 2 servings

1 Idaho potato, washed, with eyes removed

Dip
½ avocado
¼ cup chopped red onion
1 small clove garlic, minced
1 tomato, skinned and chopped
2 teaspoons coriander

Preheat oven to 375°F.

Wrap the potato in foil, stab with a fork twice, and bake until soft in the center, about 40 to 50 minutes.

To make the dip, in a blender or chopper blend the avocado, onion, garlic, tomatoes, and coriander.

Cut potato in half lengthwise, and transfer each half to a separate serving plate. Top each half with the dip. Season with a dash of sea salt and ground black pepper.

Steamed Mixed Vegetables

Makes 2 servings

1 cup fresh or frozen chopped mixed vegetables
     of your choice, such as:
     Brussels sprouts
     Broccoli
     Snow peas
     Carrots
     Cauliflower
1 teaspoon flaxseed oil
Dash of salt
Ground pepper to taste

Steam the vegetables until bold in color and crunchy; do not over-cook. Transfer to a serving plate. Drizzle with flaxseed oil. Season with salt and pepper.

Broccoli Rabe (Rapini) with Lemon

Makes 2 servings

1 tablespoon olive oil
2 cloves garlic, chopped
1 cup broccoli rabe with stems, cleaned and trimmed
Salt and pepper to taste (you can also used crushed red pepper)
Juice of 1 fresh lemon or 2 teaspoons lemon juice

Heat the olive oil and sauté the garlic briefly. Do not let the garlic turn brown. Add the broccoli rabe, salt, and pepper, then stir until just tender. Add the lemon juice. Transfer to a serving plate.

Creamed Spinach
Makes 2 servings

1 shallot, minced
1 clove garlic, minced
10 ounces frozen spinach, thawed to room temperature
¼ cup fat-free sour cream
Dash of salt
Ground black pepper or cayenne pepper to taste

Sauté the shallots and garlic until hot, about 2 minutes. Add the spinach and sauté until the liquid evaporates and the spinach is tender. Add the sour cream and salt and cook over low heat, stirring constantly, for about 3 minutes or until the sour cream liquefies. Transfer to a serving plate. Add pepper to taste.

Spicy Oven Fries
Makes 2 servings

1 russet potato, peeled and cut lengthwise into
    approximately 6 wedges
¼ teaspoon salt
½ teaspoon cayenne pepper
¼ teaspoon dried basil
½ teaspoon vegetable oil

Preheat the oven to 475°F.
Rinse the wedges and soak for 10 minutes in hot water. Remove from the water and pat dry. In a zip-top bag, combine the potatoes, salt, pepper, and basil. Turn the potato wedges until well coated.

Coat a 10- to 12-inch heavy-duty rimmed baking sheet with non-stick cooking spray.

Remove potatoes from bag and coat with ½ teaspoon vegetable oil or mist them with the oil to give them a very thin coating. Place the wedges on the prepared baking sheet and cover with heavy-duty aluminum foil. Bake for 5 minutes. Remove the foil and bake for another 15 to 20 minutes, turning potatoes over once and continuing to bake until both sides become crisp and brown.

Transfer to a serving plate.

Snacks

Honey Dipping Sauce

Makes about 4 (1 to 1 ½ teaspoon) servings

¼ cup lime juice
½ cup organic honey of your choice (choose a fragrant one)
¼ teaspoon ground nutmeg
½ teaspoon finely shredded lemon peel

In a small mixing bowl, stir the lime juice into the honey and mix until smooth. Add the nutmeg and lemon peel. Store in a glass container until ready to serve.

Banana with Peanut Butter–Honey Spread

Makes 1 serving

1 teaspoon peanut butter
½ teaspoon honey
1 small banana, peeled and sliced

In a small cup, mix the peanut butter and honey. Place the sliced banana on a serving plate. Spread the mixture over the banana.

Here we are, halfway through step 3 of my Ageless Skin–Care program. Now that you're nourishing your skin with rejuvenating food choices, you're ready to give your skin yet another boost by ramping up your activity level. You and the rest of the world have heard over and over again that exercise is key when it comes to optimum health and longevity. But did you know that exercise is also very good for your skin? You'll see results almost instantly! Turn to chapter 9 to learn more.

9

How Exercise Benefits Your Skin

Exercise is good for every organ in your body, and your skin is no exception. If you live an active lifestyle, your skin will take on a younger-looking radiance in a very short time. This reflects all the good that the exercise is also doing for internal organs such as your heart, lungs, and liver. However, I find that my patients are far more motivated to exercise when they realize that their skin will look better than it ever did when they were exhorted to get moving in order to benefit organs nobody can see! That's another reason I love being a dermatologist. I can capitalize on people's desire to look great and therefore I end up helping them improve their overall health at the same time.

HOW EXERCISE IMPROVES
YOUR SKIN

Here's what happens when you exercise and how those processes add up to younger-looking skin.

When You Are Active, Your Skin Cells Are Active

A Finnish study of middle-aged athletes showed that the athletes had noticeably fewer wrinkles than did a sedentary control group. The athletes' skin was also not as thin as the skin of the people in the control group, and it tended to be far more resilient. The researchers believe that the reason for the positive effects of exercise on aging skin is that cells in the layer where new skin is formed speed up their activity. In other words, when you get moving, your skin cells do the same!

Perspiration Is Your Skin's Own Purifier

If you exercise enough to break a sweat, you are doing your skin—and for that matter, your whole body—a big favor. Perspiration, in addition to cooling you off as it evaporates, is the body's very efficient wastes-removal system. Toxic by-products of your bodily processes, including urea and ammonia, are excreted when you sweat. Urea is also a moisturizer that helps to soften and exfoliate the skin. It is even added to many skin-care products.

In addition, sweat activates the production of sebum, a fatty substance that is your skin's built-in moisturizer. That's another reason your skin is softer and moister after a good workout. Sebum, produced by the sebaceous glands in the skin, tends to decline with age but you can maintain as peak a supply as possible if you're active. This is a tremendous benefit of exercise for your skin because sebum helps keep your skin from losing water, protects your skin from infection, and boosts your immune system. Since sebum also contributes to body odor, make sure to shower after your workout and invest in a good deodorant.

Exercise Helps Vital Nutrients Reach Your Skin

When you exercise, your blood circulation is revved up and that means that oxygen and nutrients will be delivered to your skin more efficiently. You'll find that your skin is firmer and better nourished from within. That, in turn, has a remarkable antiaging effect. Your scalp will also benefit from the increased blood circulation, and you'll have a healthier head of hair and less hair loss as a result.

Exercise Helps Reduce Stress

Exercising for at least 30 minutes daily will help reduce stress. Any reduction in stress, as you learned earlier in this book, promotes healthier and more youthful-looking skin.

You'll Get High on Your Own Hormones

Exercise promotes the release of endorphins, the mood-lifting hormones responsible for "runner's high." As you learned in chapter 5, a positive outlook goes a very long way toward erasing signs of worry and concern. When you feel good about life, you are less likely to scowl, purse your lips, and make other extreme expressions that etch lines in your face when repeated often enough. That's why pushing yourself to exercise even when you don't feel like it is so important. You may start out grumpy and overwrought, but by the end of the session you'll wonder why you ever resisted an activity that can make you feel so marvelous. When it comes to exercise, the Nike slogan, "Just do it," really fits. I truly believe that a proper exercise routine, by which I mean one that is not overly strenuous, is one of the secrets to the fountain of youth.

You'll Sleep More Soundly

Sound and restful sleep allows your skin to rejuvenate as moisture plumps it up and nutrients do their good work. If you are tossing and turning, you interrupt this natural process of renewal. Fortunately, regular exercise helps you avoid insomnia and lets you sleep deeply so that your body can nourish and hydrate your skin. Do note, however, that exercising right before bedtime is not a good idea. You'll be so invigorated that you'll need time to wind down.

THERE'S NO GOOD EXCUSE FOR NOT EXERCISING

I'm going to help you make a genuine commitment to putting exercise in your life. I hear every day in my office all the reasons that my patients have for not exercising. I've even used some of them myself in the past. So let's slay those dragons one by one and get you pumped up about the power of an active lifestyle.

I Don't Have Time to Exercise

I can certainly empathize with that statement. I'm a married working mother of two school-age children, and most of the time I actually have more than one job. I always have my busy medical practice, and I frequently add other demanding projects such as my work as a product developer, my speaking engagements, and my writing—including this book! I am passionate about all of these parts of my life and I would never choose to give any of them up. Still, I know that I owe it to myself and my family to keep myself in peak physical condition. I also believe that I deserve to treat myself well so that I'll have the very best possible skin, and that means finding time for regular exercise. One way that I do that is to walk home from work almost every day with my husband. This ensures that both of us will get some exercise and it gives us time together before we start the evening round of homework-checking and family dinnertime. We are fortunate that we work near each other. As the workday ends, we contact each other and agree what time to meet, usually on the corner of Fifty-fifth and Lexington Avenue. Then we continue to walk the rest of the way, the equivalent of about two miles, at a brisk but comfortable pace. This is a wonderful way of connecting after our busy hours apart! Another nice part for us is that since we are walking during rush hour, it would take us about the same time to get home no matter what form of transportation we used.

True, Michael and I are lucky that we live in New York City, one of the quintessential walking cities of the world. Still, I see many people here in N.Y.C. taking the subway to go just a few blocks, or hailing a cab when they could save the money and do themselves a favor by walking instead. Also, anyone can find a way to put regular walking into the day. If you live in an area where driving is the norm, try this now-classic but very useful tip: Park several blocks from your destination and also park in the farther reaches of the huge lots at suburban malls. Yes, this means a bit more time out of your busy day, but the trick is to build the walking time into your schedule. Discipline yourself not to linger before you leave the house or office. Don't read that one last e-mail or take that one last phone call or dawdle while you chat with someone. Pretend you have a plane to catch and that you really must leave at a specified time in order to make that plane.

Incidentally, all of this may seem like a lot of effort just to fit in some simple walking. However, study after study has shown that walking is a superior form of exercise that keeps you supple and young for your years. Of course that will also mean that your skin will be rejuvenated as a result. However, remember that if you are out walking during daytime, you need to apply sunscreen and wear a hat to protect your skin and scalp from UV rays.

Finally, there are plenty of ways that you can sneak exercise into your busy day. Take the stairs instead of the elevator. Stand up and stretch at your desk periodically. Rotate your ankles under your desk. None of this will cause you to break a sweat, so you won't have to take the time to shower and change clothes. Ideally, you should combine your daily exercise breaks with a real one-hour workout done three times a week. But if you miss a workout, at least you'll be getting the benefit of your daily walking, stair-climbing, and stretching.

Exercise Is Boring

The challenge is to find a form of exercise that excites and exhilarates you, or to add an element such as music to the more repetitive exercises such as the treadmill. A simple example of adding to the enjoyment of exercise is the one I just gave you about walking home in the evening with my husband. Obviously the jaunt is a whole lot more fun with him along than if I were walking solo.

Taking that concept to another level, why not enlist an exercise buddy—your best friend, your significant other, your mother, your teenager, a colleague—and plan regular exercise together. Maybe you will want to join the same gym and agree to meet at certain times, or simply get up earlier in order to meet and go for a run together.

Pearl: If you are out walking during daytime, you need to apply sunscreen and wear a hat to protect your skin and scalp from UV rays.

You'll be much less likely to skip a session if you have made a commitment to your exercise buddy!

Beyond this, remember that plenty of athletic activities are a great deal of fun and they count as excellent forms of exercise as well. I play squash, and I enjoy cross-country cycling. Believe me, neither of those activities is boring.

You might also want to join a class. You could try kick-boxing, ballroom dancing, adult ballet or tap, yoga, or karate. Another plan is to join a group such as the ones that power walk around suburban malls.

Finally, just leave the dishes in the sink and get out into the backyard with the kids or grandkids. Kick a soccer ball around. Play tag or badminton. You'll be getting fresh air, having fun with the children, and getting exercise all at the same time. The dishes can wait! Even better, you can tag-team the dishes with the family when you get back. I have found that once I let my kids know that I expected more of them in terms of setting up for dinner and cleaning up afterward, they rose to the occasion. We all benefit when the process goes more quickly, and the kids understand that.

Exercise and All the Equipment Are Expensive

Yes and no. If you follow my tips about walking more, running with a buddy, and playing with the kids, you won't be spending money on anything but a reasonably good pair of sneakers. However, if you do join a class or a gym or take up a sport, there most likely will be extra expenses. But you can check to see if there is a gym in your community, your building, or at your job that is either free or reduced in fee. Also, you can use exercise videos. Here are just a few of those that I think are particularly good:

1. Rodney Yee, *Power Yoga,* and others from him
2. Kathy Smith, *Functionally Fit,* and others from her
3. Karen Voight, *Burn and Firm,* and others from her

Also I suggest having several videos so that you can rotate them to avoid getting bored with any given routine. In any case, take a hard look at your budget and talk this over with your spouse or other family members. Building in a sum for your exercise needs is critical. It's not a luxury. It's a necessity. Doctor's orders!

I've Got a Cold

Actually, exercising in moderation when you have a cold may be good for you. Your sinuses will clear faster and you'll be boosting your immune system. However, if you have the flu or an infection such as bronchitis, you are better off taking a few days' rest. Be sure to check with your doctor, especially if you have asthma or other health concerns. Even so, don't avoid regular stretching in between desk work or naps, and make up your mind that you'll get right back to your regular exercise schedule the minute you feel better.

I'm Pregnant

You and the baby will both benefit from regular, sensible exercise throughout your pregnancy. Consult your doctor, especially if you are considered high-risk. Then look into the special exercise classes for pregnant women that are offered at many gyms and Ys around the country. There are also exercise videos for pregnant women.

I'm Not as Young as I Used to Be

All the more reason to exercise! A famous study of frail elderly patients confined to wheelchairs in a nursing home showed that the patients who used ankle weights to do quadriceps repetitions were able to walk again after only six weeks. You can improve your muscle tone at any age and with it will come all the other benefits of exercise such as improved bone density, circulation, digestion, elimination, a lift in your mood, and younger-looking skin. No, you're not going to be as vigorous an athlete as you once were, but don't give up and sit down now! Exercise is meant to be an invigorating, lifelong endeavor that keeps you in optimum health and helps you remain as youthful as possible.

COPING WITH SKIN-RELATED WORKOUT WOES

For all of its skin-rejuvenating benefits, exercise does sometimes cause temporary skin conditions you'd rather avoid. Here's how:

Extreme Flushing of the Face

Some people are much more prone to this than others. If you flush very easily, you may have rosacea (see chapter 4, page 94). Make an appointment with your dermatologist for an evaluation.

Whether or not you have rosacea or simply flush easily, you will need to give yourself some cooldown time before you return to work or social engagements. Take a warm (not hot) shower after your workout and then spend a few seconds under a cool stream of water. Remember that extremes in temperature are not good for people prone to rosacea or those who flush easily, so don't use ice-cold water. After your shower, dress and then rest for several minutes in a fairly cool area—not the overheated dressing room near the sauna at the gym! Also, look for a light foundation with a slight green component to counteract the redness of your skin. You can also use a tinted moisturizer with SPF 15 or higher. You'll soon be looking lovely again with just a fetching blush left on your cheeks.

Sweat Rash

This problem can appear as clusters of itchy red bumps or as larger hives. Sometimes called prickly heat, it is particularly common during the hot summer months. The medical term for the condition is miliaria. Some people are much more prone to miliaria than others. Research suggests that the cause of prickly heat is an increase in bacteria that live in the skin. This creates a blockage of the sweat ducts. Areas most often affected are skin folds and places where there is friction from clothing. An outbreak of prickly heat typically lasts about five to six weeks while the plugs that have been created in the sweat ducts get pushed outward. There are medical treatments that can speed up the process. Discuss them with your dermatologist. However, you can get relief from the prickly sensation by applying a topical medication such as calamine lotion. If your symptoms are extreme, your dermatologist may prescribe topical steroids such as cortisone, or topical antibiotics to fight further overgrowth of bacteria. As prevention against future outbreaks, avoid synthetic fabrics that hold in sweat, such as nylon. Look for the newer "wicking" fabrics that pull sweat away from your body. Also, be sure to shower immediately after a workout.

Acne Flare-ups

The reasons for acne eruptions after exercise are similar to those for prickly heat and the prevention tips are the same. Avoid synthetic fabrics and always—I really mean always!—shower immediately after your workout. You might even want to use an acne wash in the shower, such as one that contains salicylic acid, or one prescribed by your dermatologist. Then moisturize to make sure your skin does not end up overly dry.

Exposure to Sun, Wind, Cold, and Water

Some of the most pleasurable and beneficial forms of exercise also expose your skin to the damaging effects of the elements. If you are a skier, a swimmer, or anyone who engages in outdoor activity, you need to take every precaution to protect your skin. Slather on the sunblock and reapply every couple of hours. Use ski masks and swim goggles. Wear hats at the beach. As I've said before, I'm all for the fun of exercising in the great outdoors, but please be kind to your skin. Also, after being outside and exercising, treat your skin to a thorough cleansing and a rich moisturizer.

I hope you'll take to heart everything I've said in this chapter, and that healthful, skin-enhancing exercise will become a regular part of your life. The next chapter will teach you my unique exercise program for firming up your face and neck.

10

Firm Up
Your Face

The muscles of the face are different from muscles on other parts of the body, in that many of the former begin or end in the skin, instead of being attached to bones or tendons. Each muscle of the face has a specific action that moves the overlying skin in defined, reproducible directions. When we overuse these muscles, we not only convey emotions we may not feel quite as strongly as they may be perceived but, even worse, we end up with lines and wrinkles that make us appear older than our "girl years."

You've already heard me say that repeated extreme expressions such as frowning, grinning, and grimacing will etch lines into your face when the skin overlying the muscles stretches and doesn't snap back to its original state. Knowing that, you're probably asking yourself how I could be offering you an exercise program for the face. The answer is that there are two components. One is that with the isometric exercises I recommend, you will be contracting and releasing facial muscles in a controlled fashion that will enhance the firmness of your face.

The other is to continue the process you began in chapter 1 of learning to relax muscles you are overusing and to make expressions in a less exaggerated fashion so that they more accurately express your emotions, with the result that the wrinkles in those areas soften.

Facial muscles cannot be built up or bulked up in the same way that other muscles can because many of the important muscles of facial expression (or mimetic muscles) are attached to skin rather than to bone (see page 226, figures 10.1 and 10.2). Each muscle of the face has a specific action that moves the overlying skin in a particular defined, reproducible directions. When we overuse those muscles, we convey emotions we may not feel quite as strongly as they may be perceived, and, even worse, we end up with lines and wrinkles that make us appear older than our "girl years" and too much closer to our chronological years. However, facial muscles can be trained to lift the face up rather than pull it down. We will be working specifically with the muscles that uplift the face and avoiding those that create downward movement. Many of your uplifting muscles, such as the auricularis posterior behind your ears and the occipito frontalis under your hairline on your forehead, have no doubt atrophied from lack of use.

Most people engage only a very few facial muscles in day-to-day life. This is why I will explain how you can "find" those weakened muscles and put them to work for you in your effort to exercise your way to a natural facelift. But first, I want to explain the process of isometric exercise.

ISOMETRIC EXERCISE EXPLAINED

Isometric exercises involve contractions that generate force against resistance. A common example is pressing your hands against a brick wall. However, any contraction of a muscle that is held for several seconds and then released follows the same principle as pushing against an outside force. This is how quadriceps repetitions work. You lie on your back and straighten one leg by contracting your front

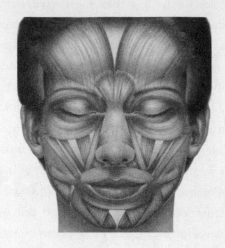

FIGURE 10.1
Muscles of facial expression.

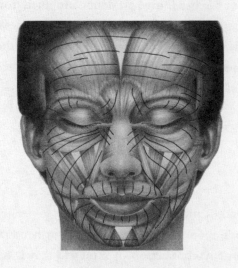

FIGURE 10.2
Facial wrinkle lines.

thigh muscle. Then you lift your leg slightly off the floor and stay there for a count of five or ten, and then relax. The facial exercises you'll be learning use this same action of contraction and release. They are done slowly and with control of the movement.

OF SYNAPSES AND SONGBIRDS

Now for that information about "finding" your atrophied muscles. Technically, this process involves creating synapses, the neural pathways from brain to muscle. A long-held belief that adults cannot manufacture new synapses was overturned not long ago by scientists who were studying how adult birds can learn new songs. The researchers discovered a process they dubbed "neurogenesis" through which the adult brain is capable of adding nerve cells and therefore learning new activity. This is very good news. Synapses permit nerve cells to communicate by converting electrical signals into chemical signals. For example, you created new synapses when you learned to ride a bike and when you learned to touch-type. At first, you had to think about every action of your muscles, but after the synapses were created, you had "muscle memory." You could then ride a bike without consciously telling your feet and body what to do, and you could type without telling your fingers what to do. If you recall, though, the process took time and repetition. The same will be true of creating synapses from your brain to your atrophied facial muscles. I hope you'll persevere, however, because the results are amazing. And just as with riding a bike or typing, once you master the facial exercises you'll be able to do them easily with no conscious effort.

DR. DAY'S FACE-FIRMING EXERCISES

Do the exercises while looking in the mirror at first. After you've perfected them and created muscle memory, you can do the exercises any time and anywhere that people won't see you and question your sanity. I recommend doing the exercises at least three but no more than five days a week. Once you have mastered them, you should be able to do all nine in about five to ten minutes total.

The Eye-Opener

1. Open your eyes as wide as possible and hold for five seconds. Relax and repeat.
2. Open your eyes wide again and roll your eyes to the right. Hold for five seconds. Relax.
3. Open your eyes wide and roll your eyes to the left. Hold for five seconds. Relax.
4. Open your eyes wide and roll your eyes upward. Hold for five seconds. Relax.
5. Open your eyes wide and roll your eyes downward. Hold for five seconds. Relax.

The Diva Look

Flare your nostrils as wide as you can, like a haughty soprano about to sing an aria. Hold for five seconds. Relax. Repeat once.

The Scream

Open your mouth as wide as possible. Hold for five seconds. Relax. Repeat once.

The Swan

Stand up straight and lengthen your neck by contracting the muscles on the side of your neck. Hold for five seconds. Relax. Repeat once.

The Frown Eliminator

Put one hand on your hairline above your eyebrows and pull gently upward. Then try to pull the muscle upward on its own. Don't be discouraged if you can't do this right away. Most people need time to "find" this muscle. When you do master the exercise, hold for five minutes. Relax. Repeat once.

The Ear Wiggle

Again, this one will probably take time to master. Start by putting your hands behind your ears and pulling gently backward. Then try to pull the muscles backward on their own. When you have succeeded, hold for five seconds. Relax. Repeat once.

The Jowl Zapper

1. Raise your chin, tilting your head as far back as possible. Hold for five seconds. Relax. Repeat once.
2. Raise your chin, tilting your head to the right. Hold for five seconds. Relax. Repeat once.
3. Raise your chin, tilting your head to the left. Hold for five seconds. Relax. Repeat once.

The Posture Perfecter

Good posture is good for all of your organs, including your skin, and it promotes good circulation.

1. While sitting down with your legs straight in front of you, sit up as straight as possible and look straight ahead.
2. Keep looking forward while you push your chin straight back. This will push your shoulders back and straighten your spine. It may feel like you are creating a double chin; that's normal.

3. Raise your arms over your head and bring them in so they touch your ears.

4. Pull down on the shoulder muscles in your back (so that your arms are no longer able to touch your ears). Hold for ten seconds. Relax. Repeat. Do this four times. Note that the muscles of your back that contribute to good posture require longer contractions and more repetitions to achieve results than do your facial muscles.

5. Stand up and repeat the contractions while also contracting your abdominal muscles.

6. You might want to try to repeat the posture part, pushing your chin back once when you are sitting in your chair at work. Take a deep breath as you go through the motions. It will give you energy and help avoid back pain, while it improves your posture. This actually makes you taller because the motion of straightening the spine can add half an inch or more to your height.

The Expression Regulator

1. Relax your face completely and close your eyes gently.

2. Let your mind go blank. You may find that a "white noise" CD will help you with this step.

3. Open your eyes, but not wide. Look at yourself in the mirror. This is your face at rest, with no expression. Note any wrinkles that are still visible. Over time as you practice my facial exercises, many of those wrinkles will be minimized when your face is at rest, and they will be even less noticeable when your face is animated. You want to remember how the face at rest feels. It is not expressionless. It is an "almost smile" with a relaxed look to the face. Once you feel it, you will see the difference and you can teach yourself to recreate it without looking in the mirror. Next time, when you are walking or listening or on the phone, you can create this expression, which will minimize the exaggerated animated movements that created the wrinkles.

This is the end of step 3 of my Ageless Skin-Care program. Take a minute to update your score on the Skin Aging Test, and make sure you're still keeping your Ageless Skin-care Regimen journal and your Three Rs journal. Now let's head into the final step of my program, when I'll help you decide whether to take advantage of state-of-the-art medical procedures that can dramatically lower your Skin Age Score without surgery.

Ageless Skin Without Surgery: Botox and Beyond

11

Wrinkle Erasers

Have you noticed that many women you encounter who have had plastic surgery look smoother, but not necessarily younger? Certainly, there is no doubt that there are times when plastic surgery is the best way to improve a person's appearance. When I feel that this is the case, I review with my patient the improvements I would hope for her to achieve. However, the goal of this book is clear. It is to make a global change in your skin, to make it look younger and healthier with life and resilience that radiate, not just to remove wrinkles. No matter how faithfully you follow the prevention advice in my Ageless Skin-Care program, certain signs of skin aging are bound to appear as the years go by. Fortunately, today we have an amazing array of state-of-the art medical procedures that can dramatically lower your Skin Age Score without surgery. An especially wonderful aspect of these treatments is that most of them do not require much in the way of down-time. You won't need to take time out of your busy life as you would if you were waiting for unsightly bruises and stitches from a facelift to heal. You can have these new nonsurgical treatments done, and tell only the people you want. Everyone else will just notice that you look great! Remember back in chapter 2 when I talked about the importance of aging in "girl years" because women in our society are still judged by their looks more than men are? With the treatments I'm going to discuss in this chapter and the next one, the improvements in your skin will look and feel completely natural. You won't have to lie about your age, because your face will do the lying for you!

That's why—as anyone who has ever glanced at the cover lines on popular magazines knows—celebrities both young and mature are benefiting these days from the rejuvenating effects of a host of new skin-enhancing procedures and treatments. The list includes the headliner, Botox, along with the newer Restylane, plus a variety of chemical and laser peels, and much more. You may have been wondering exactly how safe and effective these options are, how natural they look, and whether or not they're too pricey for anyone but the stars. The good news is that the nonsurgical medical advances in dermatology carry very minimal risk, work extremely well, and are much more affordable than plastic surgery. And as I pointed out, there's very little downtime so you can get right back to work and to your personal and social life.

Of course if you do decide to take advantage of any of the treatments and procedures I'm going to describe in detail in this chapter and the next, be certain that you choose a board-certified dermatologist or dermasurgeon with a good reputation. To clarify, dermasurgeons are dermatologists who are qualified to perform surgery, including in-office procedures. In particular, under no circumstances should you attend a "Botox party" at a private home where unlicensed people give injections of Botox obtained through uncertain channels. This warning goes double if the party involves alcohol. According to the American Academy of Dermatology, drinking during a Botox injection can cause bruising and can also affect the treatment itself since it is important not to lie down for about two to four hours after the treatment. Lying down, at least in theory, may cause the Botox to migrate away from the intended site. And alcohol or not, attempting any medical procedure anywhere except the sterile environment of a physician's office is dangerous.

However, when performed by your dermatologist or plastic surgeon, Botox injections are a reliably successful way to smooth away telltale wrinkles and take years off your face without surgery. Botox has been studied and used for over fifteen years in various parts of the body, including parts of the eyes and the muscles of the face and scalp. There have been no serious long-term side effects associated with its use by dermatologists. It is a drug consisting of a purified protein, and it is an extremely safe although temporary method of minimizing wrinkles of the face and neck. The pathway by which it acts to relax these muscles has been completely described and understood. This means that we know exactly how and why Botox exerts its effect and we can predict side effects and future uses with much greater accuracy and chance for success. So let's begin by learning about this exciting and very popular treatment.

BOTOX

Wrinkles such as "smile lines" around your mouth, "crow's-feet" at the corners of your eyes, and furrows between your brows and on your forehead are caused over time by the repeated contractions of muscles under your skin when you make facial expressions. If you have a very animated face, you may notice these "expression lines" beginning to show in your late teens or early twenties. If you have had repeated sun exposure, the collagen and elastic tissue that provide the resiliency of your skin are damaged and diminished, which accelerates the process. And by the time people reach their thirties, forties, and beyond, virtually everyone has expression lines to one degree or another.

Botox is technically safe for people as young as eighteen, but most Botox patients are at least a decade older than that. The best time to consider starting Botox treatments is when you start to see lines when your face is at rest at the end of the day, but not when you first wake

up in the morning. While you sleep, water from the increased circulation to your face when you are lying down all night plumps up your
skin. During the day as you make expressions and some of the volume
drains down toward the lower body, the plumpness disappears and lines
begin to show. This is why some people notice their legs become more
swollen as the day wears on. By evening, if you look in the mirror with
a relaxed face, you'll see the beginnings of wrinkles and furrows.

Botox treatments cost from $400 to $900, depending on how
much is used, and they are usually repeated two or three times a year
as needed.

What Is Botox?

Botox is a purified protein that is produced by the *Clostridium botulinum* bacteria, the same neurotoxin that causes a disease called botulism. There are seven different subtypes of this neurotoxin, A through
G. As far back as 1895, the microbiologist Emile-Pierre van Ermengen
recognized the possible therapeutic value of the toxin in safe doses.
There are no bacteria in the final Botox product. Though the product
of these bacteria is a dangerous toxin when found in nature, this is not
the case when it is used for medical or cosmetic purposes. Botulinum
toxin, in the hands of trained doctors, is safe and remarkably effective
in reducing or erasing lines of the face and other conditions as well.

In the 1970s, Dr. Alan B. Scott experimented with the crystallized
form of the protein to help people with afflictions such as eye twitches
and crossed eyes (strabismus). Coincidentally, he noticed that patients
who received his treatments showed a marked reduction in the wrin-
kling around their eyes. He called his drug Oculinum. In 1989, a company called Allergan bought Scott's company and changed the name of
the drug to Botox. It is derived from botulinum toxin type A. A similar drug, Reloxin, is also derived from botulinum toxin type A. It is in
the final phases of testing for FDA approval. It has been available for
years in Canada and Europe under the name Dysport. Reloxin is considered to be slightly more painful on injection than Botox. The effects

of a Reloxin treatment last for two to four months. There are also different types of botulinum toxin used outside the United States. Myobloc is used in Europe. It is derived from botulinum toxin type B.

Botox has been approved for therapeutic and for certain cosmetic purposes by the FDA for over fifteen years. Dermatologists have also developed other uses of Botox specifically for the smoothing of wrinkles on different parts of the face and neck. That's not the end of the story, though. Some patients who also suffered from migraine headaches noted that their migraines were fewer and less debilitating after they received Botox treatments, and the results often lasted six months to a year. Botox is now routinely used to alleviate migraines or tension headaches.

Another very effective use of Botox recently approved by the FDA, as discussed on page 142, is the control of hyperhidrosis, which is excessive sweating of the hands, feet, and underarms. Excessive sweating is probably one of the least discussed problems even though the condition has had a huge impact on the lives of millions of people. Most sufferers assume they are the only ones who "have it so bad" and that there is nothing to do about it, so they rarely even bring it up to their doctors.

The reason Botox was considered and tested for the purpose of treating excessive sweating is that the pathway through which Botox acts, as I mentioned, is completely understood. Scientists reviewed other organs and organ systems that utilize that pathway and experimented on ways to control hyperhidrosis, for possible side effects and adverse reactions. From this they were able to determine injection technique, which is how we make sure you get the drug only where you want it. They were also able to give a dose range that would give the best results with the fewest side effects. As a result they were able to present their data to the FDA and they received approval for the treatment of severe hyperhidrosis. This treatment has often led to life-changing improvements for many people who had been suffering for years in silence and embarrassment. People who would not enter relationships, seek higher-level jobs, or who were too embarrassed to wear any color that might show how badly they were sweating and staining their clothing are now safely and nearly instantly relieved of their anxiety and are free to pursue their goals.

How Does Botox Work?

Muscles of the face are used for facial expression and other important functions such as blinking, chewing, and moving the lips to pronounce sounds. Botox is especially useful in softening the movement of the muscles that create facial expression. However, care has to be taken not to affect the other important actions of those muscles. When administered correctly, Botox can create a soft, natural face that is more true to the feelings and expressions you mean to convey.

Specific doses of Botox are injected with a tiny needle into the muscle that is causing the wrinkle. Over the next five to seven days, the Botox effect begins. The Botox blocks nerve impulses of the muscle, which blocks the ability of the muscle to move. This causes the wrinkles in the overlying skin to soften gradually and often disappear as the expression that led to the wrinkles is also softened. (See the effects of Botox in figures 11.1 and 11.2 on page 242.) The effect lasts for about three to five months, with an average of about three months of a wrinkle-free face.

However, what's so interesting is that during the time that the Botox is working, patients can be trained not to tug at the muscles that created those extreme expressions and led to the wrinkles in the first place. In other words, although you'll need periodic injections of Botox to minimize the lines, you'll need them less often as you learn to control your wrinkle-etching muscles by yourself. If you try to overcome the effect of the Botox by insisting on continuing to make the facial expressions, you will end up recruiting other muscles and creating other wrinkles. This is one reason that Botox needs to be done carefully and why you need to learn to help yourself express in a more relaxed manner. See page 19 in chapter 2 and page 229 in chapter 10 for tips on how to do exactly that.

Botox will not affect the way your skin feels. There is absolutely no pain or numbness of the skin after Botox treatments. Also, the effects occur only in the specific muscles that have been treated. And although you may have heard scare stories from Hollywood about Botox patients having "frozen" faces that are unable to express any emotion, that is an exaggeration. There may have been a few cases of doctors or laypeople overdoing the injections, but if you are treated by a physician trained in the art of Botox injections, you'll still be able to smile, look concerned or angry, or register any other emotion on your face. Yet you won't go to the unnecessary extremes that caused your wrinkles in the first place. You will feel some resistance to the movement. This is your cue to relax and rethink the expression.

You may initially be surprised at how often you express things on your face that you don't even really feel. You are also likely to notice that people respond to you differently. In the past, the lines between your eyes may have made you look angry. Now that they are softened and you don't make that expression as often or as strongly, your whole appearance and demeanor will be changed for the better. You'll be sending positive messages to those with whom you interact instead of the negative ones associated with a scowling face. In his book *Blink*, Malcolm Gladwell explains the research on how facial expressions are tied in very closely to emotions. It may be that the expression creates or amplifies the emotion, rather than being purely a result of the emotion. This may be why so many of my patients feel so much more relaxed after their Botox treatments take effect. You just have to be careful over time not to perseverate over every minute line or expression and try to erase it. That is where you need the doctor to be able to draw the line for you and cut off your Botox supply.

The most common areas for the use of Botox are the frown lines between the eyes, the furrows of the forehead, the crow's-feet at the sides of the eyes, and creases in the neck. Botox can also be injected into specific muscles of the forehead and around and under the eyes to raise the eyebrows and create a beautiful arch. This opens the eyes and makes them appear larger. I call this the "Botox facelift," or sculpting of the face with Botox.

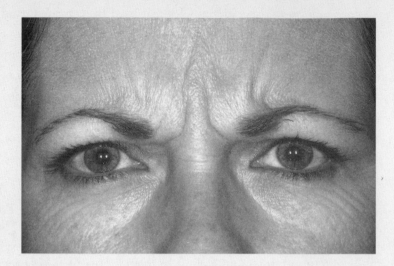

FIGURE 11.1
Furrows between the eyebrows, before Botox.

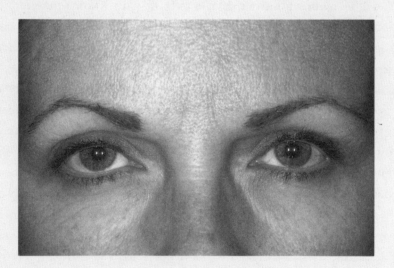

FIGURE 11.2
The furrows have been smoothed away
as a result of a Botox treatment.

Botox is also great for smoothing those bumps on the chin, and to create more of a smile in people whose mouths have a downward curve in the relaxed state.

If you're still not convinced that Botox is for you, I think this journal entry written by a patient of mine I'll call Marsha will convince you.

When I first started reading about Botox several years ago, the treatment sounded really scary. I mean, who would want to have something purposely injected into your skin that's made from the same toxin that causes botulism? Yikes! I had heard about a deadly botulism outbreak caused by people eating contaminated canned soup. Well, that was then and this is now.

Five months ago, a few weeks before my daughter's wedding, my daughter and I went together to our dermatologist, Doris J. Day, M.D., for general advice about how to improve the appearance of our skin. I don't look all that bad for my age—fifty-five—if I do say so myself. But I wanted to be the most gorgeous mother-of-the-bride I could possibly be! And my daughter is a fairly young-looking twenty-seven-year-old, but she does have some crow's-feet from too much sun.

Anyway, the doctor explained that Botox is completely safe if injected correctly and that there is no risk of disease at all. In fact, Dr. Day even told us that she uses Botox injections herself to reduce the appearance of frown lines on her forehead. When she told us that she's over forty, I couldn't believe it! She looks fantastic!

End of story: My daughter and I both got Botox injections and they were absolutely painless. Within about two days, we woke up with smoother, younger-looking faces. But unless you actually knew that we had had something done, you'd never guess. By the end of one week, my friends were telling me how impressed they were I could look so good and so calm when they knew how much effort I had been putting into this wedding. And at the wedding, people went on and on about how our happiness had made us radiant. To a certain extent that was true. But we knew the Botox was the real reason we looked so good! You should see the wedding photos!

So now my daughter and I have both decided that periodic Botox treatments will be our gift to ourselves. We deserve it! And we've found that looking good has boosted our confidence in all areas of life. It is amazing to me how much more relaxed I felt when the Botox was in effect. I would recommend Botox, in the hands of a highly trained dermatologist, to anyone who wants to look and feel years younger.

Possible Side Effects of Botox

Any medical intervention carries with it some risk of side effects. Fortunately, the possible side effects of Botox are not in any way life-threatening or permanent. Here's the list:

1. There is a small risk of bruising when Botox is injected into the forehead. The bruising is usually gone after five to seven days and clears without leaving a scar.

2. There is a very small risk of drooping of the eyelids (called ptosis) when Botox is injected around the eyes. This is temporary and can be improved with medicated eyedrops. There is also an uncommon but possible side effect called pseudo-ptosis, weakness of the forehead that makes the eyelids feel heavy and is not directly due to malfunction of the eyelids. It is uncommon and usually affects people over sixty with very heavy upper eyelids who use their forehead muscles to hold their brows up.

   In these cases, when Botox is injected into the muscles of the forehead, which are being used to hold up the brows, the forehead gets heavy and the brows appear to droop. In this case, the eyedrops don't help and you have to wait two to three months until the effect of the Botox wears off. For people with very heavy upper eyelids, Botox may only be able to correct the problem partially and Botox may even make the condition worse if too much is used in the forehead. In these cases, it may be time to consider having surgery to correct the problem. The heaviness of the eyelids may even be impairing vision. This could be why these people subconsciously go to such pains to hold the lids up.

3. When the muscles around the mouth are injected, the wrinkles are softened but there is also some associated weakness of the functions of those muscles. This can lead to mild drooling or affect your ability to whistle or make certain sounds with enthusiasm. For example, the letter "P" may be hard to pronounce. To minimize this problem, very small amounts of Botox are used because if the side effect occurs, it can last for several months. Also, it goes without saying that if you are a singer, a public speaker, an actor, or a musician who needs to make an embouchure to play a wind instrument, you should forgo this procedure and choose a soft filler instead (see below).

4. There is rarely a mild, temporary weakness of the hand when Botox is injected into the underarms or hands to control sweating. For example, you might have a little trouble opening a tight jar, but your ability to type would not be affected.

5. Although Botox is a very safe treatment, it should not be used in pregnant women or anyone with certain neurological diseases such as myasthenia gravis.

6. If you are allergic to albumin you should not have Botox injections, since human albumin is added to the Botox to help it separate from the glass vial. Albumin is a water-soluble protein that occurs in blood plasma or serum, muscle, the whites of eggs, milk, and other animal substances and in many plant tissues and fluids. If you can eat egg white, you are not allergic to albumin.

SOFT TISSUE FILLERS

If you look at the skin of a baby, or even of a teenager, the skin is supple and resilient. We now have available excellent ingredients to restore this natural resilience to the skin. Every day, patients come in completely confused about all the different treatment options available, especially collagen or other soft tissue filler and Botox. If this includes you, don't worry—you are not alone. Most people, even some very informed television anchors who have interviewed me, do not know the difference between collagen and Botox. Botox is a drug that is used to relax muscles of facial expressions in order to prevent or reduce wrinkles. Fillers like collagen are used to fill wrinkles or defects in the skin that are either still left after a Botox treatment or are in areas not appropriate for the use of Botox. There are many soft tissue fillers now available for plumping up the areas around the mouth, lips, and cheeks, and under the eyes. These fillers fall into two categories: permanent and temporary. Each has its advantages and disadvantages. The possible side effects of all fillers are essentially the same: temporary swelling and bruising, and a very small risk of infection at the treatment sites. Multiple treatments are usually necessary to achieve ideal results with intermittent maintenance treatments at varying intervals depending on the filler used in order to maintain results. Technique is critical. Make sure that you consult a qualified, experienced physician for treatment.

Temporary Fillers

The great advantage to temporary fillers over permanent fillers is that if anything goes wrong or you simply don't like the results, you are not stuck with the changes you have made. Of course the downside is that you will need to have—and pay for—treatments several times a year to keep your desired look.

Collagen Treatments: Cosmoderm, Cosmoplast

Collagen is a protein naturally found in your skin. Think of it as scaffolding that provides your skin with its firm, smooth, resilient texture. As we age and are exposed to the sun, our collagen framework breaks down and, with repeated muscle movements overlying these areas, wrinkles begin to appear. Collagen-replacement therapy restores the natural collagen support layer to your skin. Facial lines are smoothed and wrinkles are diminished. Collagen may also be used to plump up lips that have become thinner, eliminate feathery lines around your lips, and minimize the appearance of acne scars.

Two skin tests used to be required, with the second four to six weeks after the first, to determine whether or not a patient was allergic to collagen treatments. However, with the newer generations of collagen now available, such as Cosmoderm for finer lines and Cosmoplast for deeper wrinkles, skin testing is not necessary since the collagen is derived from human sources. Most people will need two or more sessions to get the best results. The treatments may need to be repeated about every four months. The injections can be painful, but topical anesthetics or nerve blocks can minimize pain.

The treatments cost about $450 and up, depending on how much is used, and I recommend two to three treatments per year.

Restylane

This soft tissue filler approved by the FDA is made of an ingredient called hyaluronic acid, which exists naturally in all living organisms. I was one of the dermatologists involved in proving the safety and efficacy of Restylane during the FDA trials. In your skin, hyaluronic acid has the ability to bind water in the tissue. However, as the amount of hyaluronic acid decreases with age, less water is bound, making the skin look older, less elastic, and less resilient. Because your body already contains the acid, injections of the substance won't be rejected and the incidence of adverse reactions is very low. If pure hyaluronic acid were injected into the skin, it would last about 24 hours. Not very satisfying. Therefore, various companies have devised techniques to stabilize the product so it will last longer in the skin. This is what separates one hyaluronic-acid product from another. So far, more than 27 million patients all over the world have been treated with hyaluronic acid–based products. As you've already learned, facial wrinkles are produced by repeated and habitual contraction of the underlying muscles during facial expression. When the facial muscles

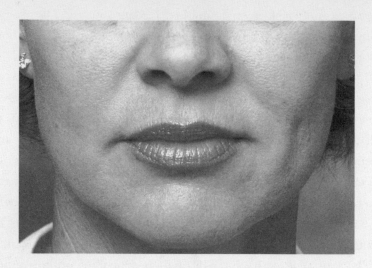

FIGURE 11.3
Folds between the nose and lips before a
Restylane treatment.

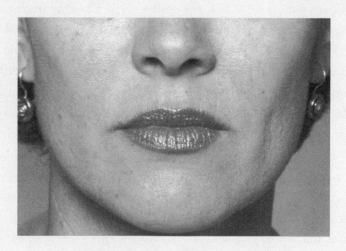

FIGURE 11.4
Folds plumped up after a Restylane treatment.

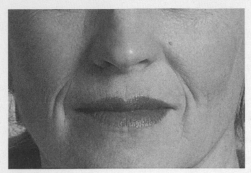

Before

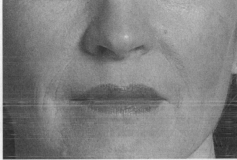

After

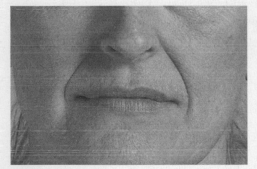

Before

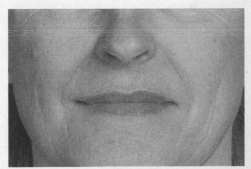

After

FIGURE 11.5
Restylane before and after.

contract, the muscles shorten without a corresponding shortening of the overlying skin, thereby producing a wrinkle. Other factors that cause aging of the skin are the thickness of the skin and the amount of underlying fat, the water content of the skin, the distribution and ratio of collagen and elastic fibers, and the biochemical changes in the connective tissue, an interstitial substance.

The function of Restylane is to add volume where the body's own hyaluronic acid has been depleted. Restylane can also be used to create extra volume in the cheeks, chin, and lips (see figures 11.3–11.5 on pages 248 and 249). A local anesthetic is generally necessary for lip augmentation. A nerve block, which is a tiny injection often done from the inside of the mouth, quickly numbs a large, local area such as the lips or the area around the mouth.

The filler, which is in the form of a gel, does cause some temporary swelling after injection that can last for 24 to 48 hours, but the swelling subsides as the gel degrades and more water binds to the site. The less concentrated the gel becomes, the more water each molecule is able to bind. Finally, the hyaluronic acid is fully degraded and reabsorbed in the same way that your body turns over your own natural hyaluronic acid. There are no harmful by-products of this process. The skin is ultimately left without any scarring or implant waste.

Restylane products are based on a hyaluronic acid from one single family of bacteria that is harmless to humans. Because it is free from animal substances and toxins, there is absolutely no risk of transmitting diseases from other species. Furthermore, there is no risk of allergic reactions in people who are allergic to animal sources such as meat, chicken, or eggs.

As an added safety measure, Restylane is also sterilized after final packaging and is therefore absolutely sterile.

Jane writes:

I had regular collagen treatments in the past and I was very happy with the results. The problem was that collagen just didn't seem to last long enough and was completely useless when I had it injected in my lips. It didn't last more than a month. When my doctor told me about Restylane I was very excited to try something new that was safe and would last longer. We talked about the options available and this was the best choice for me. I did not want something permanent injected into my face that could not be removed without surgery and scarring, so silicone and artecoll were out. We talked about the newer human forms of collagen, but my doctor explained that the studies showed that Restylane lasted longer so that was where I was going.

I was not new to injection treatments, so I knew not to have too much vitamin E or to take aspirin or other NSAIDs for about two weeks before the procedure to minimize bruising. I also had my bottle of geranium oil ready in case I did bruise, since my doctor told me that although all measures were taken to avoid bruising, the chances of a bruise could not be entirely eliminated. The geranium oil would help any bruising heal much more quickly. First the doctor marked the areas she was planning to inject and reviewed them with me while I looked in the mirror. I felt I needed it everywhere so wherever she marked looked more than reasonable to me. The initial injections to numb the areas I was having treated were painful, but the topical numbing cream softened the pain to a large degree. After that I just closed my eyes and relaxed. I felt no pain, and I let my doctor do her thing. As she moved along and finished an area, she applied a rolled-up gauze pad and had me apply pressure—to make me feel useful, she tells me—while she moved to the next area. Afterward the area was a bit swollen, but no bruises, and I could instantly see a dramatic difference. She tells me that since it is a filler, the effects are instant. My lips got really swollen, but I was not surprised or worried since I had already had collagen injections in my lips in the past and I knew the swelling would go down after a day or so. I was thrilled. No bruises, I loved the results, and I knew they would last and even improve over the next several months. The nurse gave me ice packs for a few minutes and I was off. It doesn't get better than this. I don't tell even my husband that I do this since I follow Dr. Day's motto of never point out your flaws, especially to your husband. He always thinks I look great and I like having him think I just wake up this way every day.

Treatments cost $550 and up, depending on the volume used, and last about six to nine months or more.

Hylaform and Hylaform Plus

These are hyaluronic acid produced from rooster combs. No skin testing is required. They last about as long as collagen, three to four months, and are injected in the same areas as other soft tissue fillers.

Juvéderm

FDA-approved in June 2006, it is, like Restylane, a nonanimal, nonhuman source of hyaluronic acid with results and treatment protocols similar to those of Restylane.

Occurring naturally in the body, hyaluronic acid is a natural complex sugar found in all living organisms that creates volume and elasticity in the skin. Juvéderm adds volume to facial wrinkles, such as nasolabial folds (the folds running from the sides of the bottom of the nose to the outer corners of the mouth). Botox Cosmetic works differently—by relaxing the dominant frown muscles between the eyebrows. This allows the two vertical lines between the brows, often referred to as an "11," to diminish temporarily in appearance. Like Botox, which has been available for more than sixteen years and is currently approved to treat twenty different medical conditions in more than seventy-five countries around the world, hyaluronic acid is used for multiple medical conditions, including those associated with the eye and the knee, and has been around for more than twenty years. Physicians often will use a combination of products to obtain a desired facial rejuvenation look that is natural, expressive, and fresh.

The U.S. Food and Drug Administration (FDA) approved three different formulations for Juvéderm, providing the necessary flexibility to tailor each treatment to the particular needs of the patient:

1. Juvéderm dermal filler 24HV, a highly cross-linked formulation for more versatility in the contouring and volumizing of facial wrinkles and folds.

2. Juvéderm dermal filler 30HV, a more highly cross-linked robust formulation for volumizing and correction of deeper folds and wrinkles.

3. Juvéderm dermal filler 30, a highly cross-linked formulation for subtle correction of facial wrinkles and folds.

Captique

From the makers of Hylaform, this is the newest hyaluronic-acid filler to gain FDA approval in the United States. Like Restylane, it is derived from nonhuman and nonanimal sources. However, to secure FDA approval for Captique, the makers demonstrated clinical equivalency to Hylaform, using Hylaform three-month data. The results of Captique last about three months, with similar risk for pain, swelling, and bruising as the other injectables.

Sculptra

This is a relatively newly FDA-approved filler made of a type of sugar in the alpha hydroxy acid family called poly-L-lactic acid. The same material is commonly used to make absorbable sutures—the kind that dissolves after surgery. Prior to using the product, the treating physician adds a volume of water, along with lidocaine, to the vial and lets it sit for 2 to 24 hours or longer in order for the particles to become suspended in the liquid. It is especially important to have a physician experienced in Sculptra since there is some risk of granuloma formation (small bumps in the skin). If the bumps occur, they are generally deep within the skin and are not typically visible from the surface. They are usually effectively treated with injections of cortisone directly into the bumps.

Sculptra is recommended for filling the deeper lines of the face, restoring volume and natural contour, especially on the cheeks, and enhancing the lines between the nose and the mouth and on the chin. It is also now being used to plump up the back of the hands. It should not be used in the forehead or lips since it cannot be injected deep enough at these sites and will therefore leave them looking lumpy. Several sessions are required for best results. Topical anesthetic is used as needed. Immediately after the injection there may be some swelling or bruising, but the skin will also look fuller due to the volume of water that was injected. Over the course of the first week after the treatment, it is very important to massage the areas for about 5 minutes every day, to stimulate collagen production within the skin and to minimize the risk of bumps.

The particles themselves provide some volume. However, the majority of the effect, and its longevity, are due to the particles' ability to stimulate collagen production around them. The results have been impressive and are expected to last two to four years. However, intermittent touch-ups may be needed. Sometimes another product such as Restylane or Hylaform is used as a layer over the Sculptra or for touch-ups. Sculptra may be one of the best compromises for those who would like results that last longer but who don't want a permanent filler.

Radiesse

This is an FDA-approved product, made of calcium hydroxylapatite, which is a synthetic precursor of bone, although it does not become bone when injected in the skin. It is used for the deeper lines around the mouth and fat atrophy of the cheeks. It is thought to last two to five years when used for other purposes in other parts of the body such as to help treat urinary incontinence, although studies are still under way to define more clearly how long it lasts in the skin. Results are natural.

Fascian

This product is derived from human fascia latta (fibrous connective tissue), which has been pulverized and made into a powder. It is reconstituted prior to injection and requires a relatively large bore needle to deliver the product to the desired layer of the skin. This can make the treatment more painful, usually requiring topical anesthetic along with a nerve block. It is generally used for deeper lines of the face. Results may last for one year.

Fat Transfer

This can be useful for someone who is having liposuction. Part of the fat that is suctioned can be immediately processed and injected into nearly any part of the face or hands, or it can be stored for later use. In other cases, when larger volume liposuction is not desired, or not appropriate, a smaller amount of fat can be harvested from the thigh or other part of the body, usually under local anesthesia, and used in the same manner. After the injection, there can be swelling and bruising that can last for about 5 to 10 days. The treatment lasts months to years, and is permanent in some cases. However, most people require several treatments and repeated injections over time in order to maintain results.

Permanent Fillers

These are regaining popularity as people continue to seek the longest-lasting results. The same areas are treated as with the temporary fillers. It is important to be very careful in choosing to have a treatment with a permanent filler since the results really are permanent, for better or for worse. The filler can only be removed surgically, which is bound to leave a scar. However, allergic reactions are exceedingly uncommon even for silicone when pure medical-grade silicone is used. If too much is injected in one area, that site can become lumpy, but the newest techniques of injection minimize the risk of this happening.

Artecoll

This is polymethylmethacrylate (PMMA) microspheres, a synthetic material commonly used in hip implants, bone cement, and other medical devices, which is bound to an animal form of collagen as the vehicle. Once the collagen is absorbed by the body, the Artecoll remains and offers permanent filling of the space. Small amounts are injected into the selected site over several sessions for optimal results. Two skin tests done one month apart are required to ensure you are not allergic to the collagen. Anesthetic may be required for pain management, especially of the sensitive areas around the mouth. This product is being considered by the FDA for approval.

Silicone

Studies are under way to get FDA approval for silicone as a permanent filler. While this has been a controversial ingredient, especially when women complained of a variety of problems after having breast implants, it is also becoming more popular among people who want permanent filler results. This is an "off-label" use, as silicone is not currently FDA-approved for use in the skin. There have been reports of infection and allergic reactions to silicone injections to the face, buttocks, and calves. These have come after untrained laypeople were doing the treatments using nonmedical-grade silicone. The pure medical-grade silicone used by trained physicians has virtually no risk of infection, although there are still the concerns about the outcome. I have seen silicone done well and I have seen silicone that has had less than optimal results. The results are permanent either way. Some physicians use silicone rather than any other injectable. However, while I think there are some cases in which silicone may be the right choice, I do not consider silicone to be the first choice for most of my patients, especially now that longer-lasting temporary fillers are becoming available.

As if the list of anti-aging treatments you've just learned about weren't amazing enough, the next chapter will give you the details about even more treatments designed to rejuvenate the skin. Better yet, the treatments discussed in this chapter and the next can be done together for a comprehensive regimen that gives beautiful, lasting results.

12

Rejuvenating Treatments

The procedures I'm going to discuss in this chapter can give your skin a remarkably youthful radiance. In addition, if you have any spots, scars, or discolorations on your face, these treatments can minimize those blemishes. The good news is that the treatments are safe, noninvasive, and not terribly expensive.

MESOTHERAPY

The goal of mesotherapy when used on the face is to improve some types of acne scars and to reduce wrinkles, using a combination of vitamins, minerals, and medications injected directly into a particular site. About two to four sessions may be necessary for optimal results, and there is some swelling and bruising following treatments. The therapy is also used for improving the appearance of cellulite, for spot weight reduction, and for sculpting curves. Already popular in Europe, it is slowly gaining popularity in the United States.

CHEMICAL PEELS

Chemical peels are becoming increasingly popular, and the variety of ingredients used for this purpose is increasing daily. The goal of a peel is to leave the skin smoother, more even in texture and tone, and less wrinkled. The newer combinations of peels add in antioxidants and humectants that make them stronger, yet better tolerated. Newer techniques also allow for peels of different strengths to be used at one time to permit a deeper peel on one part of the face or treatment site, and a more superficial peel at another, more delicate, site. For example, a deeper peel on the face may be combined with a lighter peel under the eyes, or a deeper peel over specific wrinkles or scars and a lighter peel for the face as a whole. This allows for an even peel on the entire treated site and a stronger effect where needed. This is what makes the treaments special and why it is so important to have an experienced physician providing the treatment.

Chemical peels speed up the natural exfoliating process in which outer layers of your skin's cells are sloughed off. Various types of acids are used to help break the chemical bonds between skin cells. In this way, the peels also accelerate the production of new cells as the skin heals and the cells below are stimulated to renew themselves. The result is a fresher, smoother, and more youthful appearance. In some states, practitioners without medical degrees are allowed to perform peels. However, you should always choose a board-certified dermatologist or plastic surgeon to perform your medium to deeper peels.

Anesthetics are not usually required for most types of peels, although you may receive mild sedation to help you relax and feel comfortable for the deeper peels. There are several different types of peels, and there are new advances in techniques in which different types of peels are used together, or in which peels are combined with laser treatments. These methods were developed to take into account the different types of skin on different parts of the face.

This is a very exciting time in terms of aesthetic products available for peels. We can get the best results with less recuperation time off from work and social activities than ever before.

Ingredients used in peels include salicylic acid, Jessner's solution, resorcinol, trichloroacetic acid, and glycolic acids, which are also referred to as fruit acids. These ingredients come in various strengths and are used in different combinations to treat various skin types and conditions of the skin. Depending on the strength of the peel, the process takes from fifteen to about forty-five minutes and may or may not cause any visible peeling. You should let your doctor know if you have had recent sun exposure or are going on vacation to a sunny area since sun exposure may affect how your skin responds to the peel. Your doctor may advise you to wait until your tan fades or until after your vacation is over before doing the peel. Taking into consideration the type of peel you are having, your doctor will also review with you medications you are taking and the products you are using on your skin to ensure that they will not interact with the peel. Some products such as retinoids may need to be temporarily discontinued about three to five days before a peel to avoid excess irritation.

Depending on the chemical used and the number of layers applied, you can end up with a superficial, medium, or deeper peel. The greater the depth of the peel, the more dramatic the results, but also the greater the risk of scarring. Superficial peels affect the upper layers, or the epidermis. Medium-depth peels penetrate to the papillary dermis, which lies immediately beneath the epidermis. The deeper peels go as far down as what is called the reticular dermis, which has a direct impact on the collagen and elastic tissue, but also therefore has the greatest risk of complications. This level of peel is generally reserved for a very small number of people with severe photoaging. Following are the most commonly performed peels and what you can expect from them:

Peels slough off the upper layers of the skin of the face, chest, back, arms, or buttocks. There is little to no downtime, and they are usually done as a series of treatments followed by maintenance treatments every few months. While these peels have a high level of safety, they are medical procedures and there is some risk of getting a deeper than expected result and the possibility of scarring, which makes it very important to be sure that a qualified aesthetic physician is performing or directly overseeing the procedure.

Glycolic Acid Peel

These fall into the family of alpha hydroxy acids (AHA), some of which are derived from fruits, which is why they are sometimes called fruit acids.

The AHAs include:

- Glycolic acid—from sugarcane
- Lactic acid—from sour milk
- Citric acid—from citrus fruit
- Malic acid—from apples
- Tartaric acid—from grapes

They are commonly used in concentrations of 8 to 5 percent in over-the-counter products. However, they are also commonly used by dermatologists in higher concentrations, up to 70 percent, as peeling agents. Layering of any particular strength of glycolic acid will not increase its strength or make it a deeper peel, as is the case with other peels that I will discuss in the chapter. Even so, the higher the concentration used, and the longer any given strength peel is left on the skin, the stronger the peel, which means the deeper the penetration and the greater the risks. Glycolic acid peels are usually recommended as a series of three to five peels, using an increased concentration, and with longer contact time, as tolerated at each subsequent visit.

These peels must be neutralized in order to stop their action when a desired end point is reached, as determined by the treating physician. Neutralization can be achieved by either flushing the area with water, or by using an alkaline solution such as 10 to 15 percent sodium bicarbonate. Often a neutralizing solution is used, and the patient is then asked to rinse the area with cool water immediately afterward to make sure the peel is terminated and all residual chemical removed.

There may be some minimal irritation or redness lasting a few hours to a few days after the procedure, especially with the higher-concentration acids. There is no actual visible peeling at the lower concentrations. However, your skin will feel firmer and more hydrated. Also, fine lines, skin discoloration, and age spots will appear diminished. Sometimes higher concentrations are used directly over brown spots or acne scars to improve their appearance. In these cases you can expect areas of redness and crusting over the next four to seven days.

This treatment can be performed on the face, chest, back, arms, buttocks, or other areas to improve such conditions as acne, thickened skin—especially on the chest and between the breasts from years of sun exposure—keratosis pilaris, a common, inherited condition where there are redness and bumps on the outer aspect of the upper arms and sometimes on the thighs and buttocks. Scarring is uncommon. Sometimes the peel—even a lighter peel—can penetrate more deeply than expected, especially if you have been using retinoids, scrubs, or other exfoliating products. Be sure to review your home regimen with your doctor to minimize the risk of havig a peel penetrate too deeply. Each peel procedure costs from $100 to $250, and I recommend one treatment every three to four weeks for two or three months, and then one treatment every three to four months as maintenance.

Lactic Acid Peel

This is another type of hydroxy acid that is more and more commonly being used for peels. It is also applied as a series, alone, or in combination with other peels or procedures.

Salicylic Acid Peel

Salicylic acid is available in over-the-counter formulations in maximal concentrations of 2 percent. In doctor's offices, concentrations of 5 to 30 percent can be used with the purpose of penetrating the epidermis (upper layers of the skin) to exfoliate the surface layer of dead skin cells and cleanse away acne-forming bacteria. Remaining surface impurities can then be removed during acne surgery. This is a process whereby blackheads are manually extracted, using special instruments designed for this purpose. Blackhead removal should not be done at home or with your fingers. Remember, your fingers are not surgical instruments.

If you try squeezing and picking at these lesions yourself, you will most likely have more redness and you'll increase the likelihood that you will have a scar at the site. That's why the in-office treatment is particularly helpful for people with acne. After application of the solution, the skin turns a frosty white and starts to have a burning sensation that lasts for about 2 minutes. The peel is self-neutralizing, with the pain diminishing and resolving once the neutralization process is complete. Over the next few days you may notice visible peeling and a tight sensation of the skin. It is important to moisturize the treated area several times over the course of the day until the peeling stops, usually in about 4 to 7 days. Your skin will be clearer, more refined, and smoother. These peels are also excellent for treatment of skin that has become discolored from years of sun exposure. Allergic reactions to salicylic acid are extremely rare, and it is considered to be an excellent tool in our peel armamentarium. However, again, it is important to have an experienced physician providing the treatment since there is salicylic acid toxicity, or salicylism, if too high a concentration is used at one time over too large an area. Your doctor will know that generally only 25 percent or less of the body should be treated at any given time. It helps to drink at least eight glasses of water in the first twelve hours after the peel since this will speed the elimination of the salicylic acid from your body. Let your doctor know if you experience any ringing in the ears or light-headedness after the peel. When done properly, and by the right person, this is an excellent gentle peel. The treatment costs about $175, and I recommend one treatment per month for two or three months, and then as needed a few times per year for maintenance.

Jessner's Peels

Jessner's solution can be used for light peels alone, or prior to a trichloroacetic acid peel. The solution contains a combination of salicylic acid, lactic acid, resorcinol, and ethanol. It has a distinct medicinal smell. As with salicylic acid peels, you can expect a good amount of exfoliation after the peel, so you might have to plan to take a few days or even weeks off for this. The solution is gently uniformly applied in layers over the desired site. The peel is applied in layers to create different levels of peel. A level-one peel usually consists of one or two layers and is a superficial peel. A level-two peel is usually achieved with two or more layers, with each successive layer creating a slightly deeper peel than the previous one. Several coats may be necessary to reach a level of peel or increase to the next level. A level-two peel is considered a medium-depth peel. Also, when Jessner's peels are combined with TCA peels, you can expect a medium-depth or deeper peel.

You can expect to feel some burning or stinging during the peel and for about fifteen minutes to half an hour after the peel is completed. Over the next one to three days, the skin feels tight and turns reddish brown, occasionally with some areas of streaking. For another two to four days after that, the skin exfoliates, revealing the refreshed, healthier skin beneath. Sometimes the exfoliation can last one to two weeks when three or more layers are applied. After the peel, it helps to apply creamy emollients many times over the course of the day. Use bland, fragrance-free moisturizers. You will also most likely be advised to avoid scrubs, masks, astringents, retinoids, alpha hydroxy acid, salicylic acid, or other topical prescription products until about two to four days after the peel has healed. In a small number of cases there is some degree of redness in several of the treated areas for several weeks after the peel. This can be more obvious after exercise, washing, or drinking alcohol, and eventually resolves without scarring.

Along with the risk of salicylic acid toxicity, there is also some risk of an allergic reaction to resorcinol and resorcinol toxicity. Patch testing behind the ear can be done two days prior to the peel to check for sensitivity to this ingredient. Also there is a very low risk of toxicity to resorcinol, depending on the amount of chemical that gets absorbed into the skin. The larger the surface area and the more layers applied, the higher the potential for toxicity. Signs of concern are dark urine, tremors, and fainting. It is more often the salicylic acid than the resorcinol that will determine how much of the body surface can be treated at any given session. It is a very popular peel, and millions have been performed over the years with excellent results. The treatment costs about $250 and up, depending on the depth of the peel and other peels concurrently applied.

Trichloroacetic Acid (TCA) Peel

Trichloroacetic acid can be used to create a superficial, medium, or deep peel, depending on the concentration of acid used and the number of layers applied. TCA is self-neutralizing and is available in concentrations of 5 to 90 percent although concentrations of 20 to 50 percent are most commonly used as a peel. Within one to three minutes of the time the acid is applied to the skin, you will feel stinging or burning as a white frost forms on the skin. The depth of penetration of the peel, or end point, is based on the intensity of the skin frost that occurs. The more layers, or the stronger the acid applied, the whiter the frost that ensues and the deeper the peel. Along with the concentration of TCA, technique and skin preparation are also very important to ensure accuracy of the peel and the desired results.

The goal is to eliminate the surface layers of dead skin, or to go deeper, to the level known as the papillary dermis. At the deeper levels, more care needs to be taken since the risk of scarring increases.

The peel is also used as a spot treatment for other skin conditions, such as acne scarring, sun spots, and warts, or on the whole face for people with extensive scarring or sun damage. Any part of the face can be treated, including the lower eyelids. The peel is also used on other parts of the body, with careful selection of concentration and layering technique to avoid scarring. The higher the concentration of the TCA, or the more a lower concentration is layered over itself, the deeper the peel, and the higher the risk of scarring. After the deeper-level TCA peels, your skin will initially appear frosty white, and then it will turn a deep red before turning dark brown about three days later and then peeling off over the next few days. Within one week to ten days, new skin that is fresh and radiant will appear. You may need to take some time off from work or make sure you don't have any major social engagements for about one week to ten days after the peel, since the process can look unsightly for that period. But ultimately, fine lines will be erased, age spots will be diminished, and collagen production will be stimulated. Your skin will look and act younger. The cost is from $250 to $750, and one or more treatments may be recommended, depending on the depth of the peel and the condition of the skin.

MICRODERMABRASION

This is a treatment in which fine, inert crystals made of aluminum oxide crystals or salt crystals are applied with varying degrees of pressure to your skin to loosen the outer layer of dead cells. The cells are then vacuumed up, using a suction device. The strength of the application and suction can be increased or decreased to achieve a more superficial or deeper effect. The result is immediately smoother-looking skin with fewer fine lines and a more even skin tone. The appearance of some types of acne scars will also be minimized. A series of five to seven treatments is required to provide the best results. The cost is from $125 to $250, and I recommend one to two treatments

per month for a series of four to six treatments followed by maintenance treatments at six- to eight-week intervals. This treatment can
be performed on the face, chest, back, arms, buttocks, or other areas
to improve such conditions as acne, thickened skin—especially on
the chest and between the breasts from years of sun exposure—and
keratosis pilaris, a common, inherited condition where there is redness and bumps on the upper arms. This condition can also occur on
the thighs and buttocks.

Allison writes:

*I started the series of microdermabrasion treatments in order to help treat
my acne and the scars that were starting to form. I found it completely
wrong that I was getting acne now that I was twenty-five years old. I was
not going to take it lying down. I should have outgrown this years ago.
Immediately after the microdermabrasion treatment my skin felt
smoother and softer, and I somehow didn't want to ruin it by picking at
it anymore. After my fifth treatment, my doctor told me I was done. She
said that I didn't need any more treatments. But as far as I was concerned, the idea of not continuing was simply not an option. I have been
going back regularly for my treatments and my skin looks great. I have
been doing it along with the gentle wave treatment. It is amazing how a
few simple treatments can make my skin look so good. My doctor does
take every opportunity to remind me to continue doing all those other
good things for my skin like using sunscreen, eating right, and exercise.
But the thing is that I want to do these things more now. I have good
skin and I want to keep it that way.*

LASER TREATMENTS

Laser is an acronym for light amplified and stimulated by the emission
of radiation. Laser light is an intense beam of light that can be used
in a variety of ways to affect the skin. The first lasers used in surgery
were designed to cut, seal, or vaporize skin tissue and blood vessels.

However, there have been many dramatic advances in the science of laser technology, with the newest generation of lasers being able to target specific elements within the skin without creating significant damage, redness, or loss of the upper layers of the skin. These newer lasers are called nonablative (no cutting) lasers, and they continue to gain in popularity as the technology improves. With new lasers coming to the market nearly every day, it is much easier to get a medical device approved by the FDA than it is to get a drug such as Restylane approved. While lasers have revolutionized our ability to offer dramatic improvements in the skin without surgery, some of the devices released in the past have had disappointing or less than optimal results, or have had to be modified for safety and/or efficacy concerns. I get calls every day from prospective and current patients who want to know if I have one particular laser or another, They've heard somewhere that it "works"—that is, makes the skin look better. They want their skin to look better, so they think, logically, from a nonprofessional point of view, that this must be a good treatment for them. No, no, no. While it is wonderful for you to be informed about the different tools available to improve your skin, it is so important for you to understand that lasers are only one of several tools that we have to treat the skin. If you see a physician who understands skin structure and function, and who is trained in laser and other cosmetic treatments, he or she will be able to review with you your appropriate treatment options and the results you can realistically expect. There are several factors that separate one laser from another, including:

- The specific energy source
- The wavelength of light emitted, and the ways the light is delivered, such as continuous wave, Q-switched, and pulsed, among others
- The range of energy-intensity level attainable, also known as fluence
- The amount of time over which the energy is delivered, also known as the pulse width

Specific lasers are often marketed to do one particular treatment or another in order to promote sales and interest on the part of the media, when existing lasers can already in fact do many, or all, of those same things. By the way, this is true for most tools, not just lasers. As a metaphor, in my kitchen I have several different pots and pans. One of them is called a spaghetti pot. However, I also use it to make some of my best soups and stews. I could use it only for one thing, but I find it just as effective to use one pot for more than just one thing. I would not really need to buy more pots and pans to do the same things I could, very effectively, do with the products I already had. It would take up a lot of space and get very expensive.

Again, it is very important to make sure you are treated by a trained dermatologist or plastic surgeon. Don't be shy about asking questions and make sure you are comfortable with the answers before you have any treatments.

This remarkable technology dramatically reverses the effects of aging and sun damage.

The most common indications for laser treatments include:

- Improvement of skin texture
- Removal of age spots ("liver" spots, sun spots, brown marks)
- Treatment of broken blood vessels (telangiectasia)
- Improvement of rosacea
- Tattoo removal
- Permanent removal of unwanted facial and body hair

Ablative/Resurfacing Lasers

These lasers are known to remove the damaged upper layers of the skin, a process that treats brown spots, wrinkles, and other signs of aging skin. As the skin recovers, the collagen is renewed and the skin looks smoother and younger. These treatments should not be done on people with a recent sunburn or suntan, or on those who have taken oral isotretinoin (an acne medication) over the previous six months. It is also important to take medications to prevent herpes virus (cold sores, fever blisters) outbreaks after the laser treatment. Even among those with no known herpes virus outbreaks, antiviral medications are usually started one day prior to the procedure and continued for 3 to 7 days after the treatment. Depending on the laser used, there is more or less downtime and more or less pain as discussed in the following sections:

Erbium: yttrium-aluminum-garnet (Er:YAG) laser redo

This laser is used for superficial skin resurfacing of the face, neck, eyelids, and hands. It has a high affinity for water absorption. This, along with its longer pulse duration, allows for ablation with less thermal damage than from the CO_2 laser (see page 270) and for a faster healing time and less redness than with the CO_2. Specific spots such as scars or wrinkles, or the entire face, can be treated with three to five or more passes of the laser at each visit to allow for greater concentration of energy at certain "problem" areas and a smooth transition between them and the surrounding skin. This makes the Er:YAG laser an excellent choice for those who have less damage or who need to have less downtime. The treatment can be repeated several times at two- to six-month intervals as needed. It is important to avoid sun exposure for at least one month prior to the treatment and one month after in order to minimize the risk of problems with pigmentation.

Prior to the procedure, the area to be treated is cleaned, and topical anesthetic is applied for 15 to 45 minutes. Immediately after the treatment, the skin will be very red and will feel hot and uncomfortable, like a strong sunburn. Over the next week, the skin will feel tight and the redness will fade as the new skin is formed. It is important to keep the skin well moisturized and to avoid scrubs, AHAs, and other possible irritants during this time. After the new skin forms in about seven days, you can start wearing makeup along with sunscreen as needed. You can also discuss the appriopriate time to restart your retinoid or usual skin care regimen, generally at about seven to ten days after the procedure.

Carbon Dioxide Laser (CO₂)

This type of laser is used for resurfacing the entire face, or for treatment of specific conditions. For example, the whole face can be treated to improve the appearance of sun-damaged skin, lines, and wrinkles, or the laser can be used for the treatment of warts, keratoses (benign and precancerous growths in the skin), and other superficial skin lesions. The target of this laser is the water in your skin, as is the case with the Er:YAG. But because it is a longer wavelength of light, it penetrates more deeply into the skin and has a stronger effect, with the accompanying higher-risk complications. The early CO_2 lasers were continuous wave lasers and were associated with excessive heat buildup and injury to surrounding skin and glands. The newer forms of CO_2 lasers allow for pulsing of the energy, which in turn allows for greater controlled targeting of the tissue, with less surrounding damage. Both types of laser are still available. The downside of treatment with this laser is that the skin can continue to look red for two to three months after the treatment. Also, some areas can lose their pigment entirely, which leaves the treated area looking a stark white. For this reason, the method is recommended only for people with lighter skin, and even then, measures are taken to avoid depigmentation of the treated areas. This treatment is usually not recommended for areas other than the face since early studies showed that scarring was a problem on other parts of the body such as the neck, back, arms, and hands. The procedure is painful, requiring topical or local anesthesia sometimes in combination with intravenous sedation or general anesthesia. After the treatment, the skin can feel hot and uncomfortable for several hours. It is important to keep the treated area clean and moisturized over the next seven to ten days and to avoid abrasive or irritating products in order to minimize the risk of infection and scarring until the new layer of skin forms. New collagen forms over the next few months, which helps reduce fine to medium-depth wrinkles and leaves the skin looking smoother and more even in color. You can generally resume your normal skin-care regimen 24 hours after completion of healing. The cost can be $1,000 or more, depending on the area treated.

Fraxel Laser

This is a new variation on the ablative laser treatment that allows for more control over the depth of laser penetration to increase the elimination of lesions, while minimizing damage to surrounding tissue. The goal is to speed healing after the procedure as compared to results with current ablative lasers, such as erbium and CO_2, and to improve the final effects. The skin can feel hot and uncomfortable after the treatment, and the treated areas can remain red for one week to 10 days afterward. There is renewed collagen formation over the next several months, and the skin is left looking smoother, more even in color, and less wrinkled.

Nonablative Lasers

The Neodinium:YAG laser targets the deeper layers of the skin directly without heating or disturbing the elements of the upper layer. The laser heats up the collagen, which stimulates it to tighten and to start to regrow. Pulsed-dye lasers target hemoglobin and some melanin within the skin. There is little to no redness or loss of the upper layers of skin, several treatments are usually required for optimal results, and the final effect is smother skin that is less red and more lustrous and luminous.

PHOTOREJUVENATION

This is a new state-of-the-art treatment for sun-damaged skin, rosacea, enlarged pores, brown spots, and broken blood vessels. What separates this from previous laser treatments is that there is no "downtime." You'll be able to go back to your normal routine immediately. This is because the light directly targets specific elements within the skin, leaving the upper layers intact. It can destroy superficial blood vessels without damaging the surrounding skin. It can target pigmented (brown) cells deep in the skin, which helps eliminate sun spots without hurting the upper layers of the skin or surrounding tissue.

The technology involves intense pulsed light, which is different from laser light in that it is a range of bands of light rather than one single wavelength and it is not unidirectional. For this reason it can simultaneously target different types of defects in the skin, although the end goal is similar: to make the skin smoother and more even in tone with more resilience. IPL technology is designed to do this very well.

Using a combination of intense pulsed light and laser technology, fine lines and wrinkles are greatly reduced. Brown spots and broken blood vessels are markedly reduced or erased. The skin has a smoother texture and a more even skin tone. An average of five to seven IPL treatments are needed for optimal results with maintenance treatments once or twice a year as necessary. The cost is $450 and up, depending on the areas being treated. No anesthetic is required since there is minimal to no pain during the treatment and no pain following treatment.

PHOTODYNAMIC THERAPY

This treatment consists of applying a solution called amino-levulinic acid (ALA) to the skin, waiting one to three hours, and then having an intense pulsed light treatment or laser treatments using a specific range of wavelengths of light. Anesthetic is generally not used. The ALA makes your skin much more sensitive to the light or laser treatment with the goal of speeding up results. These treatments are done for treatment of precancers, acne, scarring, and sun damage. There is some redness and peeling for a few days to a week after the treatment. Also the ALA makes your skin exquisitely sensitive to sunlight and bright indoor light for about 48 hours, so you have to cover up very well when going home after the treatment. You must also spend the next day or so indoors, with the blinds down and away from bright lights, or you may end up with a blistering sunburn. Sunscreen will not protect against photosensitivity reactions caused by visible light. Therefore, physical protection such as clothing and hats is a must.

THERMAGE

This technology involves using a radiofrequency source rather than a light source to heat up the deeper layers of the skin. The idea is that you see nothing from the surface, but as the deeper layers of the skin recover from the thermal injury, there is collagen tightening and renewal with essentially the effect of a gentle facelift without surgery. As the technique evolves, the energy is being better defined to target more superficial or deeper layers to minimize the risk of damage or injury to muscles, fat, nerves, and glands that sit under the treated areas. The procedure can be very painful and topical anesthesia is commonly used, sometimes along with intravenous sedation to manage the pain. Treatments cost $1,500 to $3,000, and sometimes two or more treatments are necessary, along with maintenance care over the next few years.

TITAN

The Titan, another new device available for skin tightening, uses an infrared light source to reverse the signs of aging. The heat is delivered to the deeper layers of skin, while a cooling tip protects the skin from the outside. The result of the process is collagen contraction without damaging the upper layers of the skin. As the deeper layers recover, there is collagen rebuilding, which leaves you with younger, tighter-looking skin, and only you need to know how you got it. The procedure can be performed on any areas where there is sagging skin, including the face, arm, abdomen, and thighs. Studies are still under way but results seem to be lesser or equal to those expected from thermage. Several treatments may be needed. There is some pain associated with the procedure so a topical anesthetic is used. There is minimal redness afterward. The treatment takes 30 minutes to an hour to perform, depending on the areas treated. The cost for each treatment is $1,500.

THREAD LIFT

How many times have you sat in front of the mirror, pulled your skin along your jawline back toward your ear, and thought, "If only I could have that . . ." Well now, maybe you can. The Thread Lift, sometimes called the Feather Lift or the String Lift, is slowly gaining popularity among those seeking a true lift quickly and without surgery. This procedure, which is not invasive, involves using a needle and thread with tiny barbs. The needle is inserted into the deep fat of the droopy areas of the brows, cheeks, and jawline, and the thread is looped around. As the thread is pulled back, the tiny barbs hook on to the fat, allowing the physician to lift and shape the area being treated. Once the physician is satisfied with the positioning of the treads, they are tied, knotted, and cut short so they don't show through the skin. Topical anesthesia is used as needed to minimize any discomfort from the insertion of the needles. The lifting and sculpting effects are immediate with minimal risk and minimal recovery time. You can expect some tenderness for a few weeks after the treatment. Also, for about three weeks after the procedure, you will most likely be advised to avoid rubbing the area or making extreme facial expressions. (But you've already heard me say that you shouldn't ever make extreme facial expressions!) You will also be advised to sleep on your back to avoid any trauma to the treated sites until the areas are fully healed and the threads have had ample opportunity to settle into place. It takes a few weeks for final healing, and for the sutures to settle and take final hold. There is a healing of tissue around the sutures which gives it a stronger, more established hold.

The effects of a Thread Lift are adjustable since the loops can be tightened later on as needed. This might be a good choice for those who are beginning to notice signs of drooping or sagging but who are not ready, or willing, to have invasive surgery. It is also good for those who have had plastic surgery a few years earlier and are noticing some new signs of drooping. The Thread Lift allows for a little tweaking without having more surgery. However, it is important to be realistic in your expectations. This is not a facelift. You can expect about 50 to 60 percent of the lift you might get if you had a surgical facelift. It is probably not an ideal choice for those who have heavy faces, or for those with very thin, loose skin.

The procedure takes about an hour to complete. The threads can be removed at any time if needed—for example, if one side ends up higher or lower than the other or if further tightening with new threads is deemed neccessary later on. The threads cannot be seen or felt from the skin surface. If the threads are left in place, the results are expected to last three to five years. This procedure also works very well when used with Botox, Restylane, or other fillers to maximize the results.

GENTLEWAVES LED PHOTOMODULATION

Researchers believe that this treatment uses light-emitting diodes (LEDs) as the energy source. They are sent at a low intensity to the skin, mimicking photosynthesis, the process that allows plants to use chlorophyll to convert sunlight into cellular building blocks.

GentleWaves is currently the only device available for utilizing this technology. It uses energy from LED sources, delivered in specific scanning patterns and at specific doses, specifically matched to the cellular processes of the skin that enhance the rejuvenation process. This is an especially useful procedure to do after a laser treatment, photorejuvenation, chemical peel, or microdermabrasion.

Bonuses of this procedure include:

- ⌒ No side effects, downtime, or pain
- ⌒ Remarkably safe and effective for all skin types
- ⌒ Noninvasive, nonablative, meaning that the upper layers of the skin are left intact
- ⌒ Nonthermal so there's no injury to the skin surface
- ⌒ Takes less than five minutes
- ⌒ Treats large areas such as the entire face or chest
- ⌒ No aftercare is needed

The cost is $50 to $100. I recommend eight to ten treatments done twice a week over a two-month period, and then maintenance treatments three to four times per year.

That rounds out my list of amazing nonsurgical ways to rejuvenate your skin. Certainly, I do recommend surgery in some cases, such as for people with genetic conditions like extremely large and puffy bags under the eyes or heavy eyelids. These are only two of the cases in which plastic surgery is an excellent option, and sometimes it is the best choice. Plastic surgeons play a valuable role in keeping us looking our best. My theory is that you can always do more if necessary, and that you should do everthing you can to look as healthy, natural, and youthful as possible. However, even after plastic surgery, many of the treatments I just outlined, along with my program, are still vital in order to maximize the results and to maintain them. Beyond that—and most important of all—I stongly believe that the vast majority of patients can achieve dramatic improvement in the look of their skin without ever needing a facelift.

Remember, however, that once you've had the effects of skin aging corrected with one or more of dermatology's modern miracle treatments, the responsibility to keep aging at bay is still yours. Promise me you'll follow all the advice I've given you in this book religiously from now on.

.   .   .

You've done it! You've completed my Ageless Skin-Care program. Calculate your score on the Skin Aging Test one more time. I'm sure you'll have reason to celebrate. But I'm not quite finished yet. You know by now that I am, as one of my patients said, a natural born cheerleader. I really want you to stay with my program so that you'll continue to have ageless skin as the years go by. So please take the time to read my last bit of advice in the epilogue that follows.

Epilogue:

More Than Face Value

I have dedicated my life to learning about the differences between intrinsic and extrinsic aging of the skin and to teaching that information to my patients. Now, through this book, I have been able to teach you as well. The essence of my Ageless Skin-Care program is that clear, glowing, ageless skin can only be achieved with a life approach that creates a healthy mind, a healthy body, and a healthy soul. However, my life-affirming program is not in any way arduous, nor does it make you feel deprived. On the contrary, the changes you've made as you've worked through the four steps of my program were designed to leave you feeling naturally fulfilled and eager to stay on course.

Because your skin is visible proof of the health of your whole being, when you see healthy skin in the mirror you know that you've been good to every other organ in your body as well. You also know that your mental agility and your mood have been enhanced and rejuvenated. When you follow my program, you are involved in a constant process of renewal that I call "fighting aging every step of the way."

During the time we've been together—and I do feel a bond with you even though we've never actually met—you've experienced a stunning reversal of the extrinsic aging process of your skin. I want you to promise me that you won't stop now. Every day, I have patients come into my office with skin that is old before its time. Yet there they are, going out day after day in the sun without any sun protection, going to tanning salons, eating poor diets, or always following some diet fad with the attendant inadequate calories and nutrition. Year after year, their weight yo-yos up and down. Sometimes they even smoke. Those wrinkles and age spots they are seeing have nothing to do with the normal intrinsic aging process. They are telltale signs of an unhealthy lifestyle. They are the product of decades during which the skin has been doing its best to hold up under various types of attack. I say over and over every day in my practice that I don't believe in aging gracefully. You have to fight it every step of the way. This means continuing for a lifetime to do everything you have begun doing on my Ageless Skin-Care program. It means protecting your skin from the sun, avoiding sun exposure when you can, using the right products on your skin, eating a healthy and balanced diet, exercising regularly, reducing stress, and finding ways to feel fulfilled in your life.

You're already on track. I'm proud of you. I hope you're proud of yourself. I also fervently hope that you'll stay with my program. Why not keep this book on a shelf near your bed and refer to it every so often as a kind of booster shot? If you've had a discouraging day, turn again to chapter 5, "Cleanse Your Spirit, Clear Up Your Skin." If you've overindulged in unhealthy food, don't beat yourself up. Instead, reread the advice in chapter 7, "How Eating Right Benefits Your Skin." If you've been skipping your daily Ageless Skin-care Regimen, get out your journal and start giving yourself check marks again until your good habits have been reinforced. In other words, nobody's perfect, and you may slip in various areas every now and then. When that happens, this book is there for you. Reach for it and give yourself a refresher course in any part of my program that has begun to elude you.

And, remember, I'm rooting for you. I want you not only to look your best but to feel your best now and for years and years to come. Here's to skin that reflects your dedication to keeping aging at bay. By doing so, you'll be getting much more than the face value of what you are seeing in the mirror. You'll be embracing good physical, mental, and emotional health habits that will give you every possible chance to live well and live long—and look marvelous every step of the way!

Index